KETO BREAD COOKBOOK

Delicious and easy low-carb bread recipe for healthy living.

by

GILLIAN WILLET

This document is geared towards providing exact and reliable information with regards to the topic and issue covered. The publication is sold with the idea that the publisher is not required to render accounting, officially permitted, or otherwise, qualified services. If advice is necessary, legal or professional, a practiced individual in the profession should be ordered.

- From a Declaration of Principles which was accepted and approved equally by a Committee of the American Bar Association and a Committee of Publishers and Associations.

The information provided herein is stated to be truthful and consistent, in that any liability, in terms of inattention or otherwise, by any usage or abuse of any policies, processes, or directions contained within is the solitary and utter responsibility of the recipient reader. Under no circumstances will any legal responsibility or blame be held against the

TABLE OF CONTENTS

what Is The Ketogenic Diet? 2

What Are The Different Types Of The Ketogenic Diet, And Which Is Right For You? 9

The Benefits Of The Ketogenic Diet 16

How To Reach Ketosis 25

Dangers Of The Ketogenic Diet You Need To Know ... 36

How To Optimize Your Overall Health: Good Eating Habits 49

Common Side Effects On A Keto Diet 67

How Should I Track My Carb Intake? 74

How To Start The Keto Diet 80

Keto Bread 90

    Health Benefits Of Bread 97

What Is Low Carb? 102

    The Difference Between Low-Carb Diets: High-Fat Vs. High-Protein 108

    What Can You Eat On A Low-Carb Diet? 112

    8 Benefits Of A Low-Carb Diet 120

    Is Low-Carb Bread Better For You Than Regular Bread? 134

Keto Bread Recipes 138

Basic Keto Bread Recipes 141

    Collagen Keto Bread 141

    Almond Flour Bread 145

    Low Carb Keto Bread Recipe 147

Paleo Coconut Bread.....................................149

Easy Paleo Keto Bread...............................151

Easy Cloud Bread..154

Macadamia Nut Bread................................157

Low-Carb Garlic & Herb Focaccia 159

Cauliflower Bread With Garlic & Herbs 162

Keto Bread Recipes: Flatbreads And Tortillas 164

15-Minute Grain-Free Tortillas................................164

Coconut Flour Flatbread 167

Cauliflower Tortillas 172

Buttery & Soft Skillet Flatbread 175

Keto Bread Rolls, Bagels & Buns 177

Fluffy Keto Buns......................................177

30-Minute Drop Biscuits................................179

Rosemary Keto Bagels 182

Turmeric Cauliflower Buns................................184

Low-Carb Almond Flour Biscuits..........................187

Cranberry Jalapeño "Cornbread" Muffins 189

Keto Bagels 191

Keto Bread Recipes: Pizza Crust...................193

Keto Breakfast Pizza 193

Coconut Flour Pizza Crust 195

15-Minute Stove Top Pizza Crust...................197

3-Ingredient Mini Paleo Pizza Crusts 200

Keto Bread Recipes: Dessert Breads 203

Keto Zucchini Bread With Walnuts...................203

Keto Pumpkin Bread..............................205

Low-Carb Blueberry English Muffin Bread Loaf....208

Cinnamon Almond Flour Bread............................210

Keto Chocolate Zucchini Bread............................213

Gluten-Free Cranberry Bread..................................217

SECTION 1:

KETOGENIC DIET

WHAT IS THE KETOGENIC DIET?

Have you heard of the Ketogenic Diet? What should you know about this Diet? This diet may not be as popular as some of the other diets we have commonly heard of, and that is why there are indeed so many things we have to know about this kind of diet. First of all, what is the Ketogenic Diet? This diet is derived from ketones and it is not your ordinary diet that suits everybody.

For many people, the ketogenic diet is a great option for weight loss. It is very different and allows the person on the diet to eat a diet that consists of some foods you may not expect.

So the ketogenic diet, or keto, is a diet that consists of very low carbs and high fat. How many diets are there where you can start your day off with bacon and eggs, loads of it, then follow it up with chicken wings for lunch and then steak and broccoli for dinner? That may sound too good to be true for many. Well on this diet this is a great day of eating and you will have followed the rules perfectly by following that meal plan.

This diet, as some people have claimed, should not be called a diet in the first place. Instead, it is a medical intervention as it is usually being followed by people with epilepsy, especially children.

Ketones are the substances formed when our bodies get rid of fats. What you should know about this diet is that it utilizes fats instead of our body's sugar or glucose and turns it into energy our bodies can use. The basic concept of Ketogenic diet is eating more fatty foods than carbohydrates so we can turn these fats into energy.

Fatty foods include those foods rich in margarine, butter, cheese, and other milk products, while preventing the person from eating any carbohydrate rich foods like breads, pasta, rice, and even fruits and vegetables.

Virtually all weight loss diets to varying degrees focus on either calorie reduction or the manipulation of the intake of one of the three essential macronutrients (proteins, fats, or carbohydrates) to achieve their weight loss effects.

Ketogenic diets are a group of "high-fat, moderate protein" or "high-protein moderate fat," but very low-carbohydrate diets. The term ketogenic basically refers to the increased production of ketone bodies accompanied by an elevated rate of lipolysis (fat breakdown). Ketones are the acidic by-products formed during the intermediate breakdown of "fat" into "fatty acids" by the liver.

The first sets of ketogenic diets were actually developed as far back as the early 1920s by the Johns Hopkins Pediatric Epilepsy Center and also by Dr. R.M. Wilder of the Mayo Clinic to treat children with hard to control seizures. The diets were designed to mimic the biochemical changes that occurred during periods of fasting, namely ketosis, acidosis, and dehydration. The diets involved the consumption of about 10-15 grams of carbohydrates per day, 1 gram of protein per kilogram of the bodyweight of the patient and the remaining calories were derived from fats.

Today, the promoters of ketogenic diets are strongly of the view that carbohydrates, especially the high glycemic index ones, are the major reasons why people gain weight. Carbohydrate foods are generally metabolized to produce glucose, a form of simple sugar generally regarded as the preferred energy source for the body as it is a faster burning energy.

Although the body can breakdown muscle glycogen (a mixture of glucose and water) and fat to produce energy, it however, prefers to get it from high glycemic index carbohydrates from our diets.

Of the macronutrients, carbohydrates are therefore argued to be the major cause of weight gain. This is more so because the increased intake of high glycemic index carbohydrate foods generally causes fluctuating blood sugar levels due to their fast absorption into the bloodstream and which, more often than not leads to the overproduction of insulin. This is where the problem actually starts.

Insulin is a hormone that regulates blood glucose levels and therefore controls the maintenance of the energy in/energy out equation of the body, which then rules bodyweight. Excess amounts of glucose in the bloodstream causes the excessive secretion of insulin, which leads to the storage of the excess glucose in the body as either glycogen in liver and muscle cells or as fat in fat cells.

One aim of ketogenic diets is therefore to reduce insulin production to its barest minimum by drastically reducing carbohydrate consumption while using fats and proteins to supplement the body's energy requirement.

Despite the ability of ketogenic diets to reduce insulin production, their main objective is ultimately aimed at inducing the state of ketosis. Ketosis is a condition or state in which the rate of formation of ketones produced by the breakdown of "fat" into "fatty acids" by the liver is greater than the ability of tissues to oxidize them. Ketosis is actually a secondary state of the process of lipolysis (fat breakdown) and is a general side effect of low-carbohydrate diets. Ketogenic diets are therefore favorably disposed to the encouragement and promotion of ketosis.

Prolonged periods of starvation can easily induce ketosis, but it can also be deliberately induced by making use of a low-calorie or low-carbohydrate diet through the ingestion of large amounts of either fats or proteins and drastically reduced amounts of carbohydrates. Therefore, high-fat and high-protein diets are the weight loss diets used to deliberately induce ketosis.

Essentially, ketosis is a very efficient form of energy production which does not involve the production of insulin, as the body instead burns its fat deposits for energy. Consequently, the idea of reducing carbohydrate consumption does not only reduce insulin production, but also practically forces the body to burn its fat deposits for energy, thereby making the use of ketogenic diets a very powerful way to achieve rapid weight loss.

Ketogenic diets are designed in such a way they initially force the body to exhaust its glucose supply and then finally switch to burning its fat deposits for energy. Subsequent food intake after inducing the state of ketosis are meant to keep the ketosis process running by appropriately adjusting further carbohydrate consumption to provide just the basic amount of calories needed by the body.

6

For example, the Atkins Diet, which is obviously the most popular ketogenic diet, aims to help dieters achieve what the diet calls the individual's Critical Carbohydrate Level for Maintenance (CCLM) - a carbohydrate consumption level where the dieter neither gains nor loses weight anymore.

Adequate fat intake is also essential as this enhances fat burning by the body while reducing synthesis of fatty acids in the body. Both of these actions promote fat loss. Optimal sources of fats are flaxseed oil, fish oil, avocado, olive oil, nuts and seeds.

To provide balanced nutrition, vitamins, minerals, and fiber and to promote detoxification, it is also essential to consume 3-4 cups of low carbohydrate vegetables or salad daily with one optional serving of fresh fruit daily.

It's long been established in scientific circles that blood sugar taken from food is absolutely vital for survival. Without it, a person will become sick, weak, and eventually die. However, in the past few decades, many bodybuilders have chosen to be 'guinea pigs' for their own analysis into what happens when carbohydrates - the means for bringing blood sugar into the body - are removed.

The results were twofold. First, the bodybuilders achieved new levels of muscularity and conditioning. Second, they did not die, despite the scientific belief it was impossible to maintain blood sugar levels without eating carbohydrates.

It turns out the liver creates NEW blood sugar. It takes components of lactic acid and pyruvic acid which exist in the body, and combines them with amino acids which enter the body through consumption of protein foods (or amino acid supplements). The liver forms new glycogen (blood sugar) at higher levels than it is consuming. Remember, the liver regularly breaks down glycogen as part of its normal routine.

In terms of effectiveness, ketogenic (low-carb) diets can be very beneficial for bodybuilders who are at an intermediate or advanced level, who already possess a decent amount of muscle mass. It is very hard to gain muscle while not consuming carbohydrates. Ketogenic diets are very effective because they force your body to consume fat stores for energy, instead of choosing to utilize the sugars in your blood from your daily carb consumption. There are side effects, and they are compounded greatly to cause a negative effect when the bodybuilder doesn't consume adequate fiber through supplementation or daily no-carb vegetable ingestion.

WHAT ARE THE DIFFERENT TYPES OF THE KETOGENIC DIET, AND WHICH IS RIGHT FOR YOU?

Some ketogenic (or "keto") diet devotees stay true to the diet 100 percent of the time, while others have found they need a little more carbohydrates or protein. That's inspired some to tweak the low-carb, high-fat diet to meet their own needs. As a result, several spins on the keto diet have emerged.

Kristen Kizer, RD, a registered clinical dietitian at Houston Methodist Hospital in Houston, says all of these diets have one thing in common. "A keto diet to me would be any diet that gets a body into ketosis," she says.

"Ketosis occurs when the body turns to fat as its main source of energy instead of carbohydrates," says Amy Shapiro, RD, the New York City–based founder of Real Nutrition.

Keeping the body in ketosis for extended periods of time may lead to weight loss, according to a study published in Experimental & Critical Cardiology. Ketosis is a natural metabolic state in which the body burns fat rather than carbs.

That's what motivates most people to go keto. "It's popular because in most cases it can produce very easy and effective weight loss — that's the primary reason why people start it," says Los Angeles–based Franziska Spritzler, RD, the founder of Low Carb Dietitian.

There are some other researched benefits beyond weight loss, including possibly acting as a mood stabilizer in those with bipolar disorder (per a very small study in Neurocase) and lessening epileptic seizures (according to a study published in May 2016 in Epilepsy & Behavior).

But not everyone's a fan. "For most people, going keto means jumping on the diet of the moment bandwagon," says Jackie Newgent, RDN, a culinary nutritionist in New York City and the author of The All-Natural Diabetes Cookbook. "For most, it's a fad diet that will offer temporary results."

That runs counter to Newgent's usual advice to find an eating plan you can follow for a lifetime. She also worries that reducing carbs as much as the original keto diet calls for will cut out nutrient-rich foods, like whole grains, certain veggies, and fruits.

If you're already trying a keto diet or are interested in starting one, you may be wondering which version is best for you. That depends on a few factors, including your goals, activity level, and health history.

Here, we dive into six of the most popular types of the ketogenic diet. Kizer says to keep in mind that while there are many studies involving ketosis, these variations of the diet have not yet been researched.

What Is The Strict Keto Diet And Who Uses It?

How It Works -- When people say they're on the strict version of keto, they're likely referring to the one that's been shown to help treat epilepsy. Sometimes called the "therapeutic keto diet," this is the original version of keto, which was created in the 1920s to help treat seizures, according to a study published in Current Treatment Options in Neurology.

"Strict ketosis was traditionally for those using ketosis as part of the treatment for [people with epilepsy] who were nonresponsive to medication," Kizer says.

The original study found that sticking to the keto diet for one year led to improvements for 44 percent of study participants, with another 12 percent becoming seizure-free, per a study published in June 2016 in *Practical Neurology.*

This version of the diet allows for the lowest amount of carbs (hence being the strictest). According to the *Practical Neurology* study, 90 percent of daily calories come from fat, 6 percent from protein, and just 4 percent from carbs.

It's Best for People Who ... are trying the keto diet to treat epilepsy.

Risks to Note-- The most common side effects among children who followed the diet were constipation, weight loss, and growth problems or anorexia, found as stated in the Practical Neurology study. The growth problems among children may be the result of limited protein intake, Spritzler says.

There's also a risk for developing hypercalciuria (high calcium levels in urine), kidney stones, and low blood sugar. Even though the bulk of research has been on children, adults may experience the same issues — plus possibly high cholesterol, though levels should drop once you quit the diet and start eating normally again.

Unsurprisingly, this strict version of keto also seems to be the toughest one to stick to: Research shows the modified versions of the diet have lower drop-out rates.

Thankfully, a few keto variations have been developed that are a little more flexible, and easier to stick with long-term. The traditional or standard ketogenic diet puts your body into ketosis: In this metabolic state, you burn fat (rather than carbs) as your primary fuel source, and that promotes fat loss. On a modified keto diet, your body will go in and out of ketosis, but will still shed weight and excess body fat. Check out the guide below to see how each of the four keto diet types work.

Standard ketogenic diet (SKD)

Macronutrient ratio: 75% fat,15-20% protein, 5-10% carbs

On the standard keto diet, you plan all meals and snacks around fats like avocados, butter, ghee, fatty fish and meats, olives and olive oil. You need to get about 150 grams a day of fat (the amount in nearly ¾ cup of olive oil and three times what you are likely eating now) in order to shift your metabolism so it burns fat as fuel.

At the same time, you need to slash your carbs from about 300+ grams per day to no more than 50 (which is about the amount found in just one blueberry muffin). That means sticking to leafy greens, non-starchy veggies, and low-carb fruits like berries and melon. Finally, you'll eat a moderate about of protein, which is about 90 grams per day or 30 grams at each meal (think 4 ounces of meat, fish, or poultry).

Targeted keto diet (TKD)

Macronutrient ratio: 65-70% fat, 20% protein, 10-15% carbs

The targeted keto diet is popular among athletes and active individuals who live a keto lifestyle but need more carbs. It allots an additional 20-30 grams of carbs immediately before and after workouts to allow for higher-intensity exercise and enhanced recovery. (The total carb count comes to 70-80 grams per day.) The best options include fruit, dairy or grain-based foods, or sports nutrition products. Because the additional carbs are readily burned off, they don't get stored as body fat.

Cyclical keto diet (CKD)

Macronutrient ratio: 75% fat, 15-20% protein, 5-10% carbs on keto days; 25% fat, 25% protein and 50% carbs on off days.

Keto cycling is a way to cycle in and out of ketosis while enjoying a more balanced diet on your "days off." One keto cycling approach includes five days of traditional keto diet and two non-keto days per week. Some people choose to save their off days for special occasions, holidays, birthdays, and vacations. For best results, eat wholesome carbohydrate-rich foods on your off days, including fruits, starchy veggies, dairy products, and whole grains (rather than added sugars or highly-processed fare).

High-Protein Keto Diet (HPKD)

Macronutrient ratio: 60-65% fat, 30% protein, 5-10% carb

This plan entails eating about 120 grams of protein per day (or four 4-ounce servings of meat, fish or poultry) and around 130 grams of fat per day. Carbs are still restricted to less than 10% of daily calories. Many people find this modified keto diet easier to follow, because it allows you to eat more protein and less fat than the standard keto diet. The caveat is this approach may not result in ketosis, because like carbs, protein can be converted into glucose for fuel. But the high-protein keto diet will generally result in weight loss.

How to Pick the Right Type of Keto Diet for You

It's a good idea to meet with your doctor or a registered dietitian any time you switch up your diet — whether you're on keto or another eating plan. And above all, Torchia says to listen to your body and assess your energy level and how you're feeling on the diet. "You will be your own best teacher," she says.

THE BENEFITS OF THE KETOGENIC DIET

I mentioned earlier there were numerous health benefits associated with keto for those unfamiliar; ketogenic dieting is any diet plan "low-carb" enough to switch your body into a state of producing and burning a significant amount of ketones, specifically acetoacetate (AcAc) and its derivatives beta-hydroxybutyrate (BHB) and acetone.

For those interested in background reading, I've previously written summary articles about the science of fat metabolism and ketosis here and here.

These molecules, especially AcAc and BHB, are used by the brain and other tissues for energy, and facilitate a number of health benefits I'll address below.

While the biological processes involved are extremely complex, I'd invite you to use this as the beginning of an important conversation for you and your doctor to explore together. Indeed, ketogenic dieting may or may not be appropriate for you, so please consult with your doctor before experimenting on yourself.

Focusing the brain (increased memory, cognition, clarity, and seizure control; less migraines)

Ketogenic diets were notably first used at the Mayo Clinic in the 1920s to treat children with epilepsy. While the exact mechanism of seizure prevention on a ketogenic diet is still a mystery, researchers believe it has something to do with the increased stability of neurons and up-regulation of brain mitochondria and mitochondrial enzymes.

Related to this research, some serious attention has been given to ketogenic dieting and Alzheimer's disease. Scientists have discovered increased cognition and enhanced memory in adults with impairments in these areas, and a growing body of research shows improvement at all stages of dementia. Ketosis has been shown to be effective against Parkinson's disease as well.

For a broader audience of dieters, the often-reported side effects of increased mental clarity and focus and less frequent and less intense migraines are likely related to the more stable blood sugar and altered brain chemistry occurring with this diet that also helps to improve memory and cognition.

Fighting some types of cancer

Dom D'Agostino's lab published an article in 2014 entitled "Ketone supplementation decreases tumour cell viability and prolongs survival of mice with metastatic cancer."

Here is some important background from the abstract:

Cancer cells express an abnormal metabolism characterized by increased glucose consumption owing to genetic mutations and mitochondrial dysfunction. Previous studies indicate that unlike healthy tissues, cancer cells are unable to effectively use ketone bodies for energy. Furthermore, ketones inhibit the proliferation and viability of cultured tumour cells.

Here is a good overview article of recent animal studies, which includes this 2013 article from Dom's lab:

Of course, please do not ignore your doctor's advice when it comes to cancer treatment, but—like many of the topics addressed in this article—it may be helpful for you to bring up this data during the conversation.

Preventing Heart Disease (lower blood pressure, lower triglycerides, better cholesterol profiles)

Again, related to the downstream effects of keeping blood glucose low and stable, ketogenic dieting helps keep blood pressure in check and lowers triglyceride levels.

While it may seem counterintuitive that eating a higher percentage of fat in your diet lowers triglycerides, it turns out that the consumption of excess carbs (especially fructose) is the key driver of increasing triglycerides.

And regarding HDL and LDL particles (which the body uses to move fat and cholesterol around), ketogenic dieting helps

18

raise HDL ("good cholesterol") and improve the profile of LDL ("bad cholesterol").

Decreasing inflammation (which improves acne, arthritis, eczema, psoriasis, IBS, pain, etc…)

A *Nature Medicine* article last year found a likely mechanism behind what people have known for decades: ketogenic dieting is profoundly anti-inflammatory and helps with a host of related health problems.

The researchers found that "the anti-inflammatory effects of caloric restriction or ketogenic diets may be linked to BHB-mediated inhibition of the NLRP3 inflammasome."

In other words, the key player in many inflammatory diseases is suppressed by BHB, which is one of the main ketones produced from a ketogenic diet.

Thus the implications on arthritis, acne, psoriasis, eczema, IBS, and other diseases involving inflammation and pain are significant enough that it is prompting more research attention.

Improving Energy Levels And Sleep

By day 4 or 5 on a ketogenic diet, most people report an increase in general energy levels and a lack of cravings for carbs. The mechanism here involves both a stabilization of insulin levels and readily available source of energy for our brain and body tissues.

Sleep improvements are a bit more of a mystery. Studies have shown ketogenic dieting improves sleep by decreasing REM and increasing slow-wave sleep patterns. While the exact mechanism is unclear, it likely is related to the complex biochemical shifts involving the brain's use of ketones for energy combined with other body tissues directly burning fat.

Keeping uric acid levels in check (helping kidney function and preventing gout)

The most common cause of kidney stones and gout is elevated uric acid, calcium, oxalate, and phosphorus levels as result of a complex combination of unlucky genetics, dehydration, obesity, sugar consumption (especially fructose), and eating/drinking things with a lot of purines and alcohol (e.g. meat and beer).

An important caveat is that ketogenic diet temporarily raises uric acid levels—especially when the body is dehydrated—but over time they come down:

…uric acid goes up promptly in the same time frame that ketones go up, but after 4–6 weeks, despite ketones staying up, uric acid starts to come back down. Based on this data and my clinical observations in thousands of patients, uric acid returns to or below pre-diet baseline within 6–12 weeks despite the person remaining in a state of nutritional ketosis.

Assisting gastrointestinal and gallbladder health (less heartburn and acid reflux, less risk for gallstones, improved digestion, less gas and bloating)

It is well known that grain-based foods, nightshade vegetables like potatoes and tomatoes, and sugary foods increase the likelihood of acid reflux and heartburn. Therefore, it's not surprising that eating a low-carb diet improves these symptoms and actually confronts the root problems of inflammation, bacterial issues, and autoimmune responses.

Related to this, it is known that changes in diet rapidly and reproducibly alters the human gut micro-biome. Dr. Eric Westman describes at length how a host of problems are significantly reduced or removed as a result of micro-biome changes on a ketogenic diet.

By taking away the carbohydrate in the food, I can pretty much fix every gastrointestinal problem that affects people today.

Research also shows carbs in the diet is one of the key ingredients for gallstones. Somewhat counter-intuitively, eating a sufficient amount of fat when carb intake is down helps clear out the gallbladder and keep things running smoothly to prevent gallstones from forming.

Battling a wide variety of neurologic and metabolic diseases

Kristin W. Barañano, MD, PhD and Adam L. Hartman, MD published a review in 2008 discussing the potential mechanisms of how a ketogenic diet can treat the following diseases:

Serious attention is also being given to treating Multiple Sclerosis with a ketogenic diet based on similar mechanisms.

Assisting Women's Health (increased fertility, stabilizing hormones)

An extensive review published in 2013 looked at the research and evidence of ketogenic diets enhancing fertility (long story short, it looks promising). Studies also show that Polycystic Ovary Syndrome (PCOS) can be treated effectively with low-carb dieting, which reduces or eliminates symptoms such as infrequent or prolonged menstrual periods, acne, and obesity.

Overall, keeping blood sugar levels low and stable, which results in lower overall levels of insulin in the blood, helps equilibrate and stabilize other hormone levels, especially in women. This naturally has downstream benefits on a wide variety of metabolic pathways related to insulin, such as hunger and energy utilization.

Helping the eyes (more stable vision; less risk for cataracts)

As any diabetic will tell you, it is well known that high blood sugar has a detrimental effect on eyesight and leads to an increased risk for cataracts. It's therefore not surprising that keeping blood sugar levels low improves eye and vision health, as a gazillion people have shared online, and as related diabetes research has proven.

Gaining Muscle And Improving Endurance

BHB, specifically, has been shown to promote muscle gain. Combined with tons of anecdotal evidence over the years, there is an entire movement behind bodybuilders using a ketogenic approach to gain more muscle and less fat (typically muscle gain also comes with fat gain, so there's understandable attention being given toward preventing this).

In addition, Dr. Stephen Phinney and Dr. Jeff Volek have a number of papers published about ketogenic dieting for ultra-endurance athletes. In short, once these athletes are fully fat-adapted, there is evidence to suggest mental and physical performance is significantly improved beyond a "normal" carbohydrate-rich diet.

And last, but not least, curbing diabetes, obesity, and metabolic syndrome while sparing muscle loss

Of course, there are over 160 research papers currently on Pubmed with the words "diabetes" and "ketosis" or "ketogenic" in the title alone. It's beyond clear ketogenic dieting is extremely effective for many people with both type I and type II diabetes for all the reasons discussed above related to keeping blood sugar levels and insulin in check.

In addition, recent papers within the last few years which were investigating the effect of ketogenic dieting on obesity conclude it's an extremely effective way to not only lose fat, but spare muscle loss while curbing many disorders related to obesity as well (many of which have been discussed above), including the set of symptoms and risk factors known as Metabolic Syndrome (i.e. abdominal obesity, diabetes, hypertension, and elevated cholesterol)

HOW TO REACH KETOSIS

Reaching Ketosis

Achieving ketosis is a pretty straightforward thing, but it can seem complicated and confusing with all of the information out there. Here's the bottom line on what you need to do, ordered in levels of importance:

Restrict your carbohydrates. Most people tend to only focus only on net carbs. If you want great results, limit both. Try to stay below 20g net carbs and below 35g total carbs per day.

Restrict your protein intake. Many people come over to keto from an Atkins diet and don't limit their protein. Too much protein can lead to lower levels of ketosis. Ideally for weight loss, you want to eat between 0.6g and 0.8g of protein per pound of lean body mass. To help with this, consider using the keto calculator>>>KETO CALCULATOR

Stop worrying about fat. Fat is the primary source of energy on keto – so make sure you're feeding your body enough of it. You do not lose weight on keto through starvation.

Drink water. Try to drink a gallon of water a day. Make sure you're hydrating and staying consistent with the amount of water you drink. It not only helps regulate many vital bodily functions, but it also helps control hunger levels.

Stop snacking. Weight loss tends to do better when you have fewer insulin spikes during the day. Unnecessary snacking may lead to stalls or a slow down in weight loss.

Start fasting. Fasting can be a great tool to boost ketone levels consistently throughout the day.

Start doing exercise. It's a known fact exercise is healthy. If you want to get the most out of your ketogenic diet, consider adding in 20-30 minutes of exercise a day. Even just a small walk can help regulate weight loss and blood sugar levels.

Start supplementing. Although not usually needed, supplementing can help with a ketogenic diet. Note: Always remember to be vigilant and make sure you're checking ingredients on the labels. It's too often that you will find hidden carbs in products that seem keto friendly.

Optimal Ketosis and Macros

There are so many tricks, shortcuts, and gimmicks out there on achieving optimal ketosis – I'd suggest you don't bother with any of that. Optimal ketosis can be accomplished through dietary nutrition alone (aka just eating food). You shouldn't need a magic pill to do it. Just stay strict, remain vigilant, and be focused on recording what you eat (to make sure your carb and protein intake are correct).

How to Know if You're in Ketosis

You can measure if you're in ketosis via urine or blood strips, though it's not really worth it. The urine strips are considered pretty inaccurate (they more answer the question "Am I in ketosis?"), and the blood strips are expensive (up to $5 per strip). Instead, you can use this short list of physical "symptoms" that usually let you know if you're on the right track:

Increased Urination. Keto is a natural diuretic, so you have to go to the bathroom more. Acetoacetate, a ketone body, is also excreted in urination and can lead to increased bathroom visits for beginners.

Dry Mouth. The increased urination leads to dry mouth and increased thirst. Make sure you're drinking plenty of water and replenishing your electrolytes (salt, potassium, and magnesium).

Bad Breath. Acetone is a ketone body that partially excretes in our breath. It can smell sharp like over ripe fruit, similar to nail polish remover. It's usually temporary and goes away long-term.

Reduced Hunger & Increased Energy. Usually, after you get past the "keto flu," you'll experience a much lower hunger level and a "clear" or energized mental state.

MACROS

Starting a ketogenic diet is not just about knowing the benefits, recipes and how to prepare your meals. It is also important to know their nutritional profiles and why they are an important part of a well-formulated ketogenic diet.

What are Macronutrients and Micronutrients?

Nutrients are environmental substances used for energy, growth, and bodily functions by organisms. They have two substances, macronutrients provide the bulk energy the organism's metabolic system needs to function. There are 3 macronutrients required by humans, carbohydrates, proteins, and fats.

Micronutrients provide the necessary cofactors for metabolism to be carried out. Micronutrients help build and repair tissues. It is also used to regulate body processes while macronutrients are converted to, and used for energy.

The ketogenic diet macronutrients ratio varies within the following ranges:

- ✓ 60-75% of calories from fat

- ✓ 15-30% of calories from protein

- ✓ 5-10% of calories from carbohydrates

- ✓ Most people who are in ketogenic diet don't consume more than 5% of their calories from carbohydrates.

✓ Maintenance level, also known as the Total Energy Expenditure, is a level at which you maintain a stable body weight.

✓ Maintenance level = BMR + TEA + TEF

Where:

BMR (Basal Metabolic Rate) – Amount of energy expended daily at rest and calculated using the Mifflin – St. Jeor Formula.

TEA (Thermal Effect of Activity) – Also known as the Activity level, determines additional expenditure due to moving around and exercising.

TEF (Thermal Effect of Feeding)– increase in metabolic rate when food is ingested. Protein and carbs have the highest specific dynamic action, while fat has the lowest. TEF on the ketogenic diet will be 10% on average.

Ever wondered why fat is the highest percentage of the macros consumed on a ketogenic diet? It's because good fats are really good for the body. Fats and Protein are essentials for the body's survival. Whereas there is nothing like an essential carbohydrate. There are 3 types of carbohydrates:

Simple Carbohydrate which have a simple molecule structure consisting of one to two sugar molecules. Glucose is the simplest form of carbohydrate. A good example of simple carbohydrate is table or granulated sugar. Just for clarification, not all simple carbs are bad. There are good simple carbs permissible on keto, such as certain fruits and vegetables in moderate quantities.

The second type of carbohydrate is a Complex Carbohydrate. These also have sugars, but are a more complex arrangement of chains as the sugar molecules. Some good examples of complex carbs are white rice, white sugar and pasta.

Just like the simple carbohydrates not all complex carbohydrates are bad, the unrefined foods such as some type of rice is healthy like brown rice and wholemeal flour and it should still be eaten in moderation. Although these are generally considered healthy, they do not form part of a well-formulated ketogenic diet, or lifestyle in which grains, pulses and whole wheat are foods to avoid.

The third type of carbohydrate is the Complex Fibrous Carbohydrates which are typically keto approved. These are fibrous carbs that are rich in vitamins, phytochemicals, minerals and other nutrients that our body needs. Complex fibrous carbs have low calories and are good colon-friendly foods that help clean and keep the colon healthy. A good example of these are fresh leafy vegetables and cruciferous varieties such as broccoli and cabbage.

And don't forget to watch your calorie intake, the more calories you consume. Although many people may say calories don't count on the ketogenic diet, sadly they do. Contrary to popular belief, keto is not just for weight loss, but also be used for weight gain and there are millions of people who use it for weight maintenance. You can put on weight on eating keto. So, it is important to start out right and starting out right begins with calculating the macros that support your goal.

Fat is the most calorie dense of the three macros at 9 calories per gram as opposed to 4 calories per gram of protein, or carbs. You can lose weight by eating more fat, because fat has a negligible effect of insulin levels and so the process of burning fat is uncompromised. Whereas carbohydrates and protein both have an effect on insulin (which is the fat-storing hormone) and so although they may contain less calories, they also have a greater effect on the fat metabolism. This is further proof weight gain is not just a calories-in, calories-out problem, but there is also possibly a hormonal element to take into account.

What To Eat On A Keto Diet

Keto approved carbohydrates are mostly green leafy vegetables which tend to have a lower carb count and certain nuts. Keep your diet mostly on whole simple unprocessed ingredients and foods and just sprinkle condiments to season to taste.

Here are some recommended ketogenic foods you should have at home and should be eating on a regular basis.

- ✓ Meat – choose the red meat, bacon, steak, ham, chicken and turkey. Sausages are permitted. However, beware of hidden sugars such as dextrose and maltose.

- ✓ Low-carb veggies – green veggies, onions, tomatoes, pepper, broccoli, cauliflower, etc.

- ✓ Fatty fish – tuna, salmon, mackerel and trout

- ✓ Eggs – Whole eggs.

- ✓ Butter and cream – choose grass-fed butter

- ✓ Healthy oils – Extra virgin olive oil, avocado oil, and coconut oil only.

- ✓ Avocados – Fresh guacamole!

- ✓ Cheese – unprocessed raw cheese (Cream, blue, cheddar or mozzarella)

- ✓ Condiments – Salt, pepper, healthy herbs and spices.

Foods To Avoid On Keto

Refined carbs should be treated with caution. Get your carbs from mainly leafy green vegetables. Limit your carbs to no more than 20 g per day to begin with. Avoid refined foods as they are devoid of most healthy nutrients and enzymes and often contain undesirable ingredients.

Here are some common foods to reduce or eliminate:

- ✓ Grains or starches– wheat, rice, cereal, corn, pasta, white bread, etc.

- ✓ Sugary foods – honey, maple syrup, agave, smoothies, ice cream, cakes, candy, sweeteners, soda, fruit juice, etc.

- ✓ Fruit – All fruits except small portions of berries like strawberries

- ✓ Root vegetables and tubers – potato, yam, carrots, parsnips, cassava, etc.

- ✓ Alcohol – NO beers!

- ✓ Sugar-free and diet products – they are highly processed foods and high in sugar which can affect the Ketone levels.

- ✓ Unhealthy fats – Margarine, processed vegetable and seed oils, etc.

- ✓ Beans or legumes – lentils, chickpeas, peas, etc.

- ✓ Some condiments or sauces – they usually contain sugar and unhealthy fats.

Physical Performance

People often argue that performance is affected when on a keto diet, but that's not true. Well, not in the long run. In the short-term, you may notice some small physical performance drops, but this will subside as you continue replenishing fluids, electrolytes, and adapt to the fat intake.

Many studies have been done on exercise. A study was done on trained cyclists who were on a ketogenic diet for four weeks. The results showed aerobic endurance was not compromised at all, and their muscle mass was the same as when they started.

Their bodies adapted through ketosis, limiting both glucose and glycogen stores, and used fats as the predominant energy source.

Initial Performance Drop

There was another study done on eight professional gymnasts who had the same results. Both groups were fed a strict diet of green vegetables, proteins, and high-quality fats. So, even if you are doing long bouts of cardio – a keto diet has been proven time and time again.

The only real time where ketosis can give performance loss is in exercises that needs an explosive action. If you need a little boost in your performance during these, you can "carb-up" by eating 25-50g of carbs about 30 minutes before you train.

DANGERS OF THE KETOGENIC DIET YOU NEED TO KNOW

The ketogenic diet gained popularity through the weight loss community. It's a low-carb (often 25g per day), high-fat diet triggering the body to burn fat for energy instead of carbohydrates.

With increased popularity, there has also been an increase in keto-naysayers; they think it's a dangerous fad fueled by the common desire to lose weight.

"It's unhealthy and unsustainable," they say. "How can a high-fat diet help you lose weight? It's dangerous for the heart, increases the risk of ketoacidosis, leads to poor mineral intake and electrolyte imbalance," they say. But the ketogenic diet has a well-established history of aiding in disease treatment. It has been used to help people with epilepsy (especially children) since the early 1900s, and more recently, it has been used to manage type-2 diabetes (since it lowers the need for insulin therapy).

The diet is extremely regimented and very difficult to stick to, as just one baked potato and one slice of bread could hold an entire day's worth of carbohydrates. While this is a deterrent for many, Christy Brissette, RD, a private-practice dietitian in Chicago, notes that many of her patients like the diet because of its strictness. "Some of my clients feel that the keto diet works for them because it doesn't involve any calorie counting and the rules are simple to understand," she says. "They feel they have strict parameters that can take the guesswork out of dieting."

Adherence to a keto diet food list isn't always great, though. A review published in January 2015 in the Journal of Clinical Neurology found that only 45 percent of participants were able to follow the approach as prescribed.

"The poor compliance was attributed to side effects, social isolation, and cravings," says Yawitz. And some people in the study "reported the diet simply wasn't helping them lose weight," she adds. Brissette agrees with this line of thinking. "In my opinion, the keto diet isn't sustainable and takes the joy and fun out of eating," she says.

As you can see, there are many potential benefits and side effects of the ketogenic diet. Here, we'll delve into 11 potential dangers of the keto diet that any beginners considering the approach need to know.

1. Serious Muscle Loss Is a Possible Side Effect of Keto

"Muscle loss on the ketogenic diet is an ongoing area of research," says Edwina Clark, RD, a dietitian in private practice in San Francisco. "Small studies suggest that people on the ketogenic diet lose muscle even when they continue resistance training. This may be related to the fact protein alone is less effective for muscle building than protein and carbohydrates together after exercise."

Meanwhile, according to a small study published in March 2018 in the journal *Sports*, people following the keto diet for three months lost about the same amount of body fat and had about the same muscle mass changes as people following normal diets. Yet the folks on keto did lose more leg muscle.

"Loss of muscle mass as we age has a number of serious consequences," notes Clark. "Muscle is metabolically active and helps boost daily energy expenditure and mitigate age-related weight gain." Losing muscle mass can also decrease functional strength and heighten the risk of falls, notes Clark. Falls are the top cause of death from injury in older populations, according to the Institute of Medicine Division of Health Promotion and Disease Prevention.

2. Keto Can Put Stress on the Kidneys and Possibly Give You Kidney Stones

Kidney stones are a well-noted potential side effect of the ketogenic diet. Research published in the Journal of Child Neurology observed that among children following the keto diet as a treatment for epilepsy, 13 out of 195 subjects developed kidney stones. Children supplementing with potassium citrate in the study noticed a decreased likelihood of kidney stones. Speak with your healthcare practitioner about supplementing if kidney stones are a concern.

"If you're going to do keto, there's a better and a worse way to do it," says Yawitz. "Loading your plate with meats, and especially processed meats, may increase your risk for kidney stones and gout," which is a painful type of arthritis. "High intake of animal proteins makes your urine more acidic and increases calcium and uric acid levels. This combination makes you more susceptible to kidney stones, while high uric acid can increase your risk for gout," adds Yawitz.

And the ketogenic diet can be dangerous for people with kidney disease, as people with kidney disease need to follow an individualized diet as prescribed by their doctor. According to Davita Kidney Care, people with kidney disease often need to consume a low-protein diet, which may not align with the type of keto you're following.

3. The Possibility of Low Blood Sugar Can Make Keto Risky for People With Diabetes

Carbohydrates help control blood sugar levels, which are of particular importance for people with diabetes. A study published in May 2018 in the journal Diabetic Medicine shows that while a keto diet may help control HbA1c levels (a two- to three-month average of blood sugar levels), the diet may also cause episodes of hypoglycemia, which is a dangerous drop in blood sugar. Echoing many registered dietitians, the Lincoln, Nebraska–based sports dietitian Angie Asche, RD, says she is "hesitant to recommend a ketogenic diet for individuals with type 1 diabetes."

The same goes for people with type 2 diabetes. While some preliminary research suggests the keto diet may be safe and effective for certain people with type 2 diabetes, there's still the risk for low blood sugar, especially for those on insulin, and the keto diet omits certain food groups known to benefit those with this disease.

For example, a study published in September 2016 in the journal *Nutrients* highlights the importance of whole grains for helping to control weight, as well as episodes of high blood sugar. Whole grains are off-limits on the ketogenic diet.

The best course of action is to proceed with caution and consult a professional before diving in. "If you have a medical condition or are on medications, you should always consult with your doctor before beginning a ketogenic diet," Asche says.

4. Because It's Hard to Follow, Keto Can Lead to Yo-yo Dieting

"Rapid, significant weight loss is a common side effect of the keto diet because of the water losses that occur as carbohydrate stores are depleted," says Clark. In a study in the *American Journal of Clinical Nutrition*, obese men following a modified version of the ketogenic diet, with high protein and low carbs, lost about 14 pounds in one month, compared with the control group, which lost about 10 pounds on a high-protein, medium-carb diet.

Jalali says people following the diet has the best chance of keeping the weight off if they stay on it long term. And that's not always easy to accomplish. The weight may come back if you go back to your regular eating habits. And regaining weight may lead to other negative effects. "Chronic yo-yo dieting appears to increase abdominal fat accumulation and diabetes risk," notes Clark.

"Studies have shown the ability to stick to a diet is more important for long-term success than the type of diet that's followed," says Yawitz. "Keto is incredibly restrictive and is particularly tough for those who have frequent social engagements or are prone to carb cravings." The Mediterranean diet allows you to eat carbs, like as many fruits and veggies as you want, along with whole grains. Not to mention, the Mediterranean diet has been linked to a number of other health benefits, including a lower risk of Alzheimer's and Parkinson's disease, certain types of cancer, and heart disease, according to the Mayo Clinic.

5. The Ketogenic Diet Can Lead to Dehydration and a Loss of Electrolytes

"Suddenly and drastically reducing carbohydrates sets your body up for a double whammy of sorts," says Yawitz. "The brain's favorite fuel is glucose, which is most easily created from carbohydrates. In very-low-carb diets, the brain has to adjust to using ketones from digested fats for energy. To add to this discomfort, your kidneys release more electrolytes as insulin levels fall."

Additionally, your total body water decreases as carbohydrates become depleted on a keto diet, notes Clark. The result? What's known as the keto flu, which could cause constipation, nausea, headache, fatigue, irritability, cramps, and other symptoms. Don't fret, though: Many of these symptoms are short term and should last only a few days to weeks. Make sure to drink plenty of water to help your body cope with these symptoms. And call your doctor if symptoms — especially nausea — are prolonged, advises Yawitz.

6. Because Keto Severely Limits Carbs, You May Develop Nutrient Deficiencies

When carbohydrate intake is low, fiber consumption tends to be low, too. "This doesn't come as a surprise when you consider fruits, whole grains, and starchy vegetables are decreased in your diet," says Asche. This can lead to one especially uncomfortable side effect (more on that below).

Another possible nutrient deficiency: potassium, a mineral important for both electrolyte balance and blood pressure control, notes MedlinePlus. "Inadequate intake of potassium is likely when consumption of fruits and starchy vegetables are decreased," says Asche. She recommends adding lower-carb sources of potassium to the diet, including avocado and spinach — as well as lower-carb sources of fiber, such as chia seeds and flaxseed (be sure to enjoy ground flaxseed for the best health benefits).

7. Bowel Problems, Such as Constipation, Are Also Common on Keto

Let's talk about a keto side effect that may not be so sexy: constipation. "Many of the richest sources of fiber, like beans, fruit, and whole grains are restricted on the ketogenic diet," says Clark. "As a result, ketogenic eaters miss out on the benefits of fiber-rich diet such as regular laxation and microbiome support. The microbiome has been implicated in everything from immune function to mental health." Indeed, in a long-term study in the *Journal of Pediatrics* in April 2015, constipation was noted as a very common side effect in children receiving ketogenic diets for epilepsy treatment.

In addition to constipation, diarrhea can crop up as a side effect of the keto diet — especially in the first few weeks of following it. "Some people have difficulty digesting large amounts of dietary fat, which can lead to greasy diarrhea," notes Yawitz.

Other causes of diarrhea on the keto diet include consuming a diet low in fiber (fiber helps ward off diarrhea by bulking up stool) and eating processed low-carb foods like shakes and bars that may contain sugar alcohols. These sugar alcohols can ferment in the gut and cause gastrointestinal discomfort.

Yawitz suggests limiting foods labeled "sugar free" if you're prone to gas or diarrhea when you eat them. And you may want to gradually adjust your carbs downward and your fats upward. "Also build your diet around [naturally] high-fiber, low-carb foods like avocado and nonstarchy vegetables such as broccoli, cauliflower, and asparagus," she says. Other keto-friendly ways to get more fiber include chia seeds, almonds, and coconut.

8. As Your Body Adjusts to Ketosis, You'll Probably Have Bad Breath

Considered a symptom of the keto flu, your breath on this diet often smells fruity at first. This is because acetone is a by-product of ketosis and is eliminated mostly through the lungs and the breath, according to a study in the journal *International Journal of Environmental Research and Public Health* in February 2014.

Acetone is a type of ketone known for having a fruity aroma in smaller concentrations. "It's hard to say exactly how long it will last as it depends on the person, but it's common for someone to experience this side effect for a few weeks," says Asche.

9. Your Period on Keto Might Undergo Some Changes

"Periods may become irregular or completely stop on the keto diet," says Yawitz. "This is more due to rapid weight loss than the diet itself and happens because of drops in gonadotropin-releasing hormone, follicle-stimulating hormone, luteinizing hormone, estrogen, and progesterone."

Long-term disruption of menstruation can bring on serious side effects, including low bone density. "This is because estrogen is very important to bone health," says Yawitz. "Studies have also found prolonged menstrual irregularity to increase risk for cardiovascular disease, depression, anxiety, and sexual dysfunction. It's important to contact your ob-gyn if your cycles become irregular or if you stop having periods."

But wait, there's one loophole. Have polycystic ovary syndrome (PCOS)? Then the keto diet may help regulate your periods. "Women with PCOS have high insulin levels, which cause sex hormone imbalances," notes Yawitz. In a small study published in the journal *Nutrition & Metabolism*, subjects with PCOS following a ketogenic diet for six months noted improvements in their menstrual cycles — and a small number of women became pregnant, overcoming previous infertility obstacles. "This study was very small, so we can't make recommendations for all women with PCOS based on its findings," says Yawitz. "And really, any diet that leads to weight loss should help in PCOS."

10. Keto Could Cause Your Blood Sodium to Dip

"When you start the keto diet, you lose sodium and other electrolytes in the urine due to reductions in insulin," says Yawitz. "This is a major contributor to symptoms of keto flu." So it's important to replenish sodium through the diet, especially if you exercise or sweat a lot. "This can help ward off more serious side effects seen with long-term sodium deficiencies," says Yawitz. These include lethargy and confusion — and in extreme cases, seizures, coma, and death, according to the Mayo Clinic.

11. Keto May Lead to High Cholesterol and an Increased Risk for Heart Disease

The ketogenic diet doesn't put a cap on saturated fat or even trans fats. The latter are fats you should always avoid. Read ingredient labels and avoid any food with partially hydrogenated oils, aka trans fats. These fats heighten your LDL ("bad") cholesterol levels and lower your HDL ("good") cholesterol levels. They also raise your risk of heart disease and stroke, according to the American Heart Association.

"Certainly, the quality of fat counts," says Yawitz. "There's a big difference nutritionally between bacon and almonds. As much as possible, people set on the keto diet should emphasize plant-based, unsaturated fats like nuts, seeds, olive oil, and avocado, which have even been shown to protect the heart."

If you have high cholesterol or other risk factors for heart disease, you should speak with your doctor before beginning the keto diet. This is because the diet may — but doesn't have to — include large amounts of saturated fat. Some studies have shown increases in cholesterol and triglycerides in people following the diet, while other research reveals the keto diet may actually decrease heart disease risk as well as saturated fat intake.

What Everyone Should Do Before They Attempt the Keto Diet

The bottom line? If you're thinking about trying the ketogenic diet, run it by your doctor first — regardless of any preexisting health conditions. And consult a registered dietitian nutritionist (find one at EatRight.org) to find a nutrition professional who can work with you to create a meal plan you can stick to.

People with kidney disease or a history of disordered eating should avoid the diet, and people with type 1 diabetes may want to avoid it, as well. If you have risk factors for heart disease, you'll want to speak with your doctor before considering the diet.

HOW TO OPTIMIZE YOUR OVERALL HEALTH: GOOD EATING HABITS

In the first of this new series "How To Optimize Your Overall Health" is a compilation of good eating habits to help you maximize the health you gain from what goes into your mouth. Proper nutrition helps form the foundation that supports your overall livelihood. In other words, when you eat the best, your body becomes its best.

The human body thrives and can exceed your expectations when fuelled properly. It's worth noting that the benefits of healthy eating habits reach far beyond vanity and appearance. Without adequate nutrition, you welcome unwanted guests such as illness, chronic disease and weight gain. Luckily, the solution is simple: Make these changes in your daily life and watch your body evolve into its most functional, beautiful, dynamic, balanced and healthy self.

Minimize Processed Foods

In this age, you're surrounded by quick, fast and convenient food options. That convenience typically means you're getting nutrient-depleted, empty-calorie foods. These easily accessible foods may fill your stomach, but they are hindering your health—especially when consumed on a regular basis.

The occasional splurge is reasonable and will not overhaul all of your healthy eating efforts. However, the key is to keep those indulgences to 10-20% of the time. The other 80-90% of the time, stay on track with foods that truly equip your body to keep up its "housework."

To be clear, processed foods include anything that has undergone complex processing steps. Additives, artificial colouring and other chemical agents are often added during these processes. A few examples of processed foods to avoid are:

Refined grains: cereals, baked goods

Refined Sugar & Artificial Sweeteners: candy, corn syrup, soda

Packaged meats

That's not to say you need to avoid packaged foods all of the time, at all costs. Rather, get familiar with reading ingredient lists and deciphering what is in your food. When buying packaged foods, look for these things on the packaging:

- No Additives

- No Artificial Flavouring

- No Artificial Colouring

- No Preservatives

- No Added Sugar

- Organic

- Grown without pesticides

- Non-GMO

- Raw

- Free Range, Cage Free, Wild Caught, Hormone Free (when buying eggs and meat)

Not every packaged food you come across will boast every one of those specifications. To keep your shopping mentality simple, think:

- Organic

- Short Ingredient List with recognizable ingredients

It's important to realize that organic, nutrient-rife foods are becoming just as accessible as processed, junk food options. Thus, all you need to do to buy these foods is head to a different isle of your grocery store. More grocery stores are integrating a natural or organic section, helping consumers more easily access good quality foods.

Supporting and purchasing from your local farmers market is another way to get your hands on high quality, organic food. Not only are you supporting your local agriculture and the families that work hard for it, but you are buying food that organically nourishes your body.

Stop Drinking Soda

If drinking soda is one of your guilty (or not so guilty) pleasures, you should pause to think about what you're really putting in your body each time you take a sip. Soft drinks — especially diet ones — are among the worst things you can put in your body. Drinking them will make you sick, fat and stupid..therefore you should put and end to it, and am very sorry to break it to you.. These sugar-filled (or artificially sweetened) beverages are nutritionally stripped and chock full of damaging preservatives and chemicals. The only purpose of these foods is to temporarily satisfy a caffeine or sugar craving.

Your body was not meant to ingest food like this. Your body needs whole, real foods with a high nutritional value to thrive. Morph this detrimental soda habit into these healthy eating habits that will actually contribute to your overall wellness:

Kombucha:

This effervescent, fermented tea beverage is becoming increasingly more accessible in your local grocery or health food store. The symbiotic culture of bacteria and yeast (as unappetizing as it sounds) and probiotics give this drink its digestive benefits. Your stomach requires an adequate amount of good bacteria in order to facilitate assimilation and absorption of nutrients.

Thus, drinking kombucha daily can help optimize your gut health as well as minimize stomach aches and discomfort. Swapping out soda for this healthy drink is one of a few good eating habits that can make large strides in your body's vitality.

Probiotic Drinks:

Similar to kombucha, probiotic drinks contain digestive aids called probiotics that balance your gut's bacteria levels. The difference between kombucha and probiotic drinks is:

Kombucha is brewed and fermented with tea, sugar, fruit juice and a SCOBY disc (a symbiotic culture of bacteria and yeast).

Probiotic drinks are often the same ingredients, sans tea. They boast similar nutritional benefits and can be consumed interchangeably.

Herbal Tea:

Consuming herbal teas, such as chamomile or peppermint, is another good health habit to form. These drinks can be used to help decrease your caffeine intake, or simply for their health benefits. Chamomile naturally aids the liver, while peppermint naturally decreases inflammation in the body.

Don't Overdo Caffeine

What's not to love about the morning coffee or afternoon tea ritual? Grinding the beans, smelling the robust aroma of the freshly brewed coffee and pairing it with breakfast is a beloved past time of many. Likewise, sharing an afternoon glass of tea with your loved ones provides comfort and togetherness. The problem lies not in drinking the coffee/tea, rather in drinking too much of it.

It's important to perhaps limit your coffee & tea drinking to your favourite times. In other words, don't mindlessly drink caffeine throughout the entire day. Try to limit your consumption to 1-2 cups of coffee in the morning, if you're a coffee drinker, and similarly if you're a tea drinker. Or, perhaps you enjoy both. Then, you can sensibly have a cup of each in a day's time and keep your caffeine intake at bay.

As with every other dietary concern, too much of something leads to imbalance in your body. In regards to this popular drink, too much consumption can cause your adrenal glands to kick it into overdrive. This becomes very taxing on your endocrine system. Ultimately, you are setting yourself up for some hormonal imbalances–which affect merely every bodily process.

In addition, too much caffeine can wreak havoc on your sleep patterns. Know that caffeine is a vasoconstrictors; essentially meaning you feel stimulated and temporarily energized after consuming it. Thus, drinking caffeinated drinks close to bed time can hinder your ability to fall asleep.

Eat Whole, Real Foods

Organic food

In the ever-growing world of convenient and packaged foods, it's easy to forget one of the greatest, most effective healthy habits is eating whole, real foods in their natural form–not packaged, not powdered, not pasteurized. You should aim to eat them as close to the source as possible. In other words, buy local produce and prepare it in ways that your body will find easy to assimilate and absorb.

Often times, packaged food products are so broken down, isolated and manipulated that your body can no longer seek their real and complete nutritional value. This doesn't mean there is no place in your diet for foods sold in a package. Rather, they should be eaten in moderation–not as the mainstay.

To receive all the nutritional benefits of nature's bounty, aim to do a lot of shopping in the "outline" of your grocery store. In other words, stay out of the isles that contain baked goods, chips, boxed meals, condiments, etc. Your focal point should be on high-quality, organic foods like vegetables, fruit, seeds, nuts, beans, grass-fed meat, free-range eggs and wild-caught fish. These foods are rife with nutrients and will provide your body with the necessary nutrients it needs.

Look to eat these healthy, organic foods 80-90 percent of the time. It's important to note that eating a flawless, perfect diet is not always realistic. Don't inflict guilt on yourself if you stray from these nutritious foods 10-20% of the time. That small amount will not break your healthy lifestyle. It's about finding balance and making good, healthful choices the majority of the time.

Get Enough of Each Macro-Nutrient

When venturing out on a mission to buy a cart full of healthy & organic food, remember that you need to get adequate amounts of each macronutrient to help your body thrive. Macronutrient is the overarching word to describe carbohydrates, proteins and fats. Contrary to what many fad diets have made you believe, your body needs all three of these components in order to function correctly.

If you relate to numbers, keep the 40-40-20 ratio in your mind. This means your daily intake should be comprised of approximately 40% carbohydrates, 40% protein and 20% fat on a given day. There's no need to measure and no need to obsess over these numbers. They are meant to simply provide you with the idea that you need all three, with a little less fat than protein and carbohydrates.

A great way to achieve this is to be conscientious of what you're shopping for. If you have a cart full of fruit and juice (all sugar), then it's time to take inventory of what that means for your diet. Create a grocery list that helps you cover all of your bases.

Some healthy sources of protein include:

- Beans (green, cannellini, black, pinto, lima)

- Nuts (almonds, cashews, brazil nuts, macadamia nuts)

- Seeds (chia, hemp, flax)

- Free-range eggs

- Grass-fed beef

- Wild-caught fish

- Healthy sources of carbohydrates include:

- Fruit (apples, berries, pineapple, oranges, grapefruit, nectarines–just to name a few)

- Raw Honey (in small amounts)

- Raw Agave Nectar (in small amounts)

- Healthy sources of fat include:

- Raw coconut oil

- Other plant based oils (olive, grapeseed, avocado)

- Ghee

- Avocado

- Seeds (chia, hemp, flax)

Aim to have a few items from each macro category in your grocery basket to insure that you're satisfying your body's needs.

Drink Enough Water

The human body is comprised mostly of water. Water is the means by which your body rids itself of toxic build up from the foods you consume and the pollutants you absorb. This vital fluid helps facilitate merely all of the complex processes within your body.

Implementing this method of staying hydrated is a helpful healthy eating habit for a few key reasons:

- Helps maintain a clear complexion

- Regulates and facilitates digestion

- Prevents dehydration

- Curbs cravings

- Boosts energy levels; leaves you feeling rejuvenated

- Prevents urinary tract infections

- Aids weight loss

- Encourages Detoxification

- Prevents headaches

A good rule of thumb is to drink water before you're thirsty. Don't wait until you feel depleted to take a few gulps. It's also helpful to bring a water bottle with you to work, school and/or on your commute. This will insure you stay adequately hydrated and feeling revitalized.

Focus your meals around Vegetables

Take a look at a traditional meal and you're likely to find a few side dishes focused around a hunk of protein like chicken or beef. The content on a plate like this isn't the problem, but the ratios can be altered a bit to up your veggie intake. Refocusing your meals around vegetables is another one of these simple, good health habits that can make a big difference for your overall weight, health and balanced lifestyle.

Making vegetables the focus of your meals does several positive things for your diet:

- Insures that you meet your daily vegetables intake

- Increases your nutrient intake

- Reduces the caloric content of your meal

- Helps you to get acquainted with new vegetables

When you implement all of these daily rituals, you are helping yourself form healthy habits for life. When you establish these habits and form a new, healthful routine, you set yourself up for many years of vitality and energetic living.

Making small changes one week at a time will help you be successful in taking on your healthy strategy. This will also increase the likelihood you stick with this new lifestyle. Feeling inundated can lead to abandoning the whole plan altogether. For instance, your first month of healthy habit forming could look like this:

Week 1: Cut out the majority of the processed foods & soda you're consuming.

Week 2: Develop a macro-balanced grocery shopping list.

Week 3: Integrate lots of organic fruits and vegetables

Week 4: Leave yourself a reminder to grab a bottle of water on the way to work

And continue to integrate a new habit with each coming week. If you feel confident enough, you can create these new habits within a week's time, or even all at once

What Happens To My Body

Your body is used to the simple routine of breaking down carbohydrates and using them as energy. Over time the body has built up an arsenal of enzymes ready for this process and only has a few enzymes for dealing with fats – mostly to store them.

All of a sudden your body has to deal with the lack of glucose and increase in fats, which means building up a new supply of enzymes. As your body becomes induced into a ketogenic state, your body will naturally use what's left of your glucose.

This means your body will be depleted of glycogen in the muscles – which can cause a lack of energy and general lethargy.

Transition Period

In the first week, many people report headaches, mental fogginess, dizziness, and aggravation. Most of the time, this is the result of your electrolytes being flushed out, as ketosis has a diuretic effect. Make sure you drink plenty of water and keep your sodium intake up.

In fact, you should go overboard with the salt – salt everything! Sodium will help with water retention and help replenish the electrolytes. For most, this temporary groggy feeling is the biggest danger you're going to face. It's called the "Keto Flu."

Keto Flu – This flu is very common for people starting out on the ketogenic diet. They experience discomfort such as headaches, nausea, fatigue, cramps, 'brain-fog', increased hunger, sleep issues, heart palpitations and constipation. Everyone experiences the keto-flu in different ways. The symptoms vary by person and it is a normal part of the pre-adaptation phase when your body is not yet used to utilising ketones for fuel.

It can take a few weeks or so to pass, but it does pass and in the meantime, can be managed by balancing electrolytes and adding sea salt to food and adding mineral supplements. Keto flu is a very common experience for new ketoers, but it often goes away after just a few days – and there are ways to minimize or even eliminate it. When transitioning to keto, you may feel some slight discomfort including fatigue, headache, nausea, cramps, etc.

There are a few reasons for the keto flu, but the two primary ones are:

Keto is a diuretic. You tend to go to the bathroom more to urinate, which attributes to a loss of both electrolytes and water in your body. You can usually help combat this by either drinking broth made from bouillon cubes or Powerade Zero and by increasing your water intake. Mainly, you want to replenish your depleted electrolytes.

You're transitioning. Your body is equipped to process a high intake of carbs and a lower intake of fat. Your body needs to create enzymes to be able to do this. In the transitional period, the brain may run low on energy which can lead to grogginess, nausea, and headaches. If you're having a large problem with this, you can choose to reduce carb intake gradually.

After increasing water intake and replacing electrolytes, it should relieve most all the symptoms of Keto Flu. For an average person starting a ketogenic diet, eating 20-30g of net carbs a day, the entire adaptation process will take about 4-5 days. My advice is to cut your carbs to fewer than 15g to ensure you are well on your way into ketosis within one week. If you are experiencing any more keto flu symptoms, double check your electrolyte intake and adjust.

You may notice that if you're an avid gym goer, you lost some strength and endurance. A temporary decrease in physical performance is typical. Once your body becomes keto-adapted, your body will be able to fully utilize fat as its primary source of energy.

Ketoacidosis – It's a very life-threatening condition where ketones in the blood surge to levels exceeding 7 mMol and can result in death and requires urgent medical care. This is a risk for Type 1 diabetics with impaired pancreatic function. Ketoacidosis is not a risk for normal healthy adults including Type 2 diabetics who are able to produce trace amounts of insulin to maintains insulin levels below danger levels.

How To Maintain A Healthy Lifestyle

Being healthy should be part of your overall lifestyle, not just a New Year's resolution. Living a healthy lifestyle can help prevent chronic diseases and long-term illnesses. Feeling good about yourself and taking care of your health are important for your self-esteem and self-image. Maintain a healthy lifestyle by doing what is right for your body.

Step 1

Maintain a healthy weight. Determine whether you are overweight by checking your body mass index. If you are overweight, it can lead to a higher risk of chronic disease such as cardiovascular disease, diabetes, stroke and certain cancers.

Step 2

Stick with healthy food from each food group. This means staying away from food high in saturated fats, sodium and added sugars. Eat more whole grains, lean proteins such as chicken or legumes and beans, low-fat or non-fat dairy, and increase your fruits and vegetables.

Step 3

Visit your doctor for an annual physical exam. Depending on your age, certain lab tests and screenings, such as mammograms, colonoscopies and heart tests, are necessary. Stay up to date on your health screenings to identify whether there are medical problems to address.

Step 4

Make sure your relationships are positive and healthy ones. Surround yourself with people who support you and who you feel good around. Your partner in life, friends and others who are in your life should respect you. If you find yourself in an unhealthy relationship, take steps to improve it or move on.

Step 5

Engage in physical activity for at least 30 minutes every day. Take an exercise class, join the gym or just take a brisk walk outside. Making the time for physical activity is a necessity and not a luxury.

Step 6

Know when and how to de-stress. Taking care of your mental health is just as important as taking care of your physical health. Make sure that you have positive ways of dealing with stressors in your life. This might be exercising, meditating, yoga or just doing deep-breathing exercises. If stress becomes so severe that it is interfering with your sleep or ability to cope, talk to your doctor or a counsellor.

Step 7

Do not smoke. Smoking can cause preventable diseases such as lung cancer and other cancers. Stay away from second-hand smoke, since this can also be hazardous to your health.

COMMON SIDE EFFECTS ON A KETO DIET

Although the adverse effects related to the ketogenic diet are generally less severe than those of anticonvulsant medications used to treat epilepsy, individuals following the diet may experience a number of undesirable effects.

Although major side effects are rare on low-carbohydrate diets —even after three years of sticking to the diet — we must understand what this kind of diet does to the body. With this knowledge, we can prevent or relieve almost all potential side effects and feel better on a low-carbohydrate diet than we did while eating more carbohydrates.

Here are a few of the most common side effects that I have come across when people first start keto. Frequently the issues relate to dehydration or lack of micronutrients (vitamins) in the body.

Make sure you're drinking enough water (close to a gallon a day) and eating foods with good sources of micronutrients.

Cramps

Cramps (and more specifically leg cramps) are a pretty common thing when starting a ketogenic diet. It usually occurrs in the morning or at night, but it's a pretty minor issue overall. It's a sign there's a lack of minerals, specifically magnesium, in the body.

Make sure to drink plenty of fluids and eat salt on your food. Doing so can help reduce the loss of magnesium and get rid of the issue.

If the problem persists, try supplementing with a magnesium supplement.

Constipation problems

The most common cause of constipation is dehydration. A simple solution is to increase water intake and try to get as close to a gallon a day as possible.

Making sure vegetables have some fiber in them will also usually help. Getting in some good quality fiber from non-starchy vegetables can solve this problem. Though if that's not enough, usually psyllium husk powder will work or taking a probiotic.

Heart Palpitations

When transitioning to keto, you may notice your heart is beating both faster and harder. It's pretty standard, so don't worry about it.

If the problem persists, make sure you're drinking plenty of fluids and eating enough salt. Typically this is sufficient to get rid of the problem right away. Though if the issue persists, it may be worth taking a potassium supplement once a day.

Reduced Physical Performance

You may see some limitations on your performance when you first begin a keto diet, but it's usually just from your body adapting to using fat. As your body shifts to using fat for energy, all of your strength and endurance will return to normal.

If you still notice problems with performance, you may see benefits from in taking carbs prior to your workout (or cycling carbs).

Less Common Side Effects On A Keto Diet

These are some of the lesser common problems that I am e-mailed about on a semi-consistent basis. Many of these problems also relate to hydration and micronutrients, so make sure you are drinking plenty of water and replenishing electrolytes.

Breastfeeding

There are mixed and matched studies on keto and breastfeeding, though nothing is well researched at the current moment. Right now it's understood that ketogenic diets are typically healthy to do while breastfeeding.

It's suggested to add in 30-50g extra carbs from fruit when breastfeeding to help the body produce milk. You may also have to add in extra calories.

Breastfeeding on ketogenic diet

Specifically, 300-500 calories worth of extra fat is needed to help with milk production. You should always contact medical professionals for advice.

Hair Loss

If you're experiencing hair loss within five months of starting a ketogenic diet, it's most likely temporary. You can take a multivitamin and do what you normally do.

Though hair loss is very uncommon on keto, you can minimize it by making sure you're not restricting calories too far and making sure you get 8 hours of sleep a night.

Increased Cholesterol

Usually, it's a good thing! Many studies point toward cholesterol elevation when doing a low-carb, ketogenic diet.

Higher cholesterol is generally due to HDL (the good cholesterol) increasing – lowering your chance of heart disease. You may see increased triglyceride counts, but that's very common in people losing weight. These increases will subside as weight loss normalizes.

There's a small percent of people who experience raised LDL cholesterol as well. These elevated levels are usually fine – though harder to test. The dangers of LDL cholesterol come from the size and density, which are shown to be very healthy on keto.

Gallstones

Of the few studies done on keto and gallstones, most people have either improved or cured gallstone problems. The only downside is that many reported an increase in discomfort when starting out on low-carb. If you stick with it, you should notice a vast improvement.

Another common question relating to gallstones is "Can I start keto if I have had my gallbladder removed?" The answer is yes.

You may want to increase your fat gradually to allow your system some time to get used to it.

Indigestion

Generally speaking, switching to keto gets rid of indigestion and heartburn. Keep in mind some people see increased attacks when they're first starting out.

If you're experiencing problems, it may be best to limit the amount of fat you intake; gradually increasing the amount you have per day over a two-week period.

Keto Rash

There's no real scientific reasoning/explanation behind why some people start to itch when they start keto. There's just a handful of experiences that people have written about, and so I'm basing my answer on what I've read.

From anecdotes, it's most likely irritation from the acetone that is excreted in sweat (it's why you may experience bad breath).

It's worth looking into better clothing options for absorbing or wicking sweat from your body. It's also worth showering right after activity that causes you to sweat.

If it's a lasting issue that is causing problems, you may want to consider upping your carbs or changing exercise plans.

Troubleshooting Further

Sometimes there's issues or problems that aren't covered in this guide. There are many other articles on the site, so make sure to search. If you're having trouble with a specific question, we have a very helpful community on the website too!

How much weight will I lose?

A: The amount of weight you lose is entirely dependent on you. Obviously adding exercise to your regimen will speed up your weight loss. Cutting out things that are common "stall" causes is also a good thing. Artificial sweeteners, dairy, wheat products and by-products (wheat gluten, wheat flours, and anything with an identifiable wheat product in it).

Water weight loss is common when you first start a low carb diet. Ketosis has a diuretic effect to it that can cause many pounds of weight loss in only a few days. While I hate being the bearer of bad news, this isn't fat. But on a side (and more positive) note, that shows your body is starting to adjust itself into a fat burning machine!

HOW SHOULD I TRACK MY CARB INTAKE?

A: The most common ways to track your carbs is through MyFitnessPal and their mobile app. You cannot track net carbs on the app, although you can track your total carb intake and your total fibre intake. To get your net carbs, just subtract your total fiber intake from your total carb intake.

Others choose to use Fat Secret, which is an app I am unfamiliar with, although I do know you can track your net carbs. The choice is entirely up to you and up to your free will to decide.

I cheated and want to get back on keto. How do I do that?

A: First take a breath; it's not the end of the world. You may find that your weight goes up temporarily as your body retains water. You may also find the scale goes down pretty quickly when you lose that water. If you see the scale fluctuating, please keep in mind there's a biological reason for it.

Pick yourself up, get back on track, and stay strict to keep cravings down. If you're having trouble with the planning aspect, you may want to consider looking into our Keto Academy Program.

I'm not losing any more weight. Now what?

A: Many things can cause a slowdown in weight loss: stress, lack of sleep, exercise, hormonal changes, and alcohol use among other things are factors. Weight loss will not always be a linear process, either. We have fluctuations in water that happen every day.

On average people will lose 1-2 lbs. a week, but that doesn't mean the scale will drop consistently. Take measurements as well as tracking your weight via scale, as often there can be changes in size but no change on the scale. If you're still experiencing problems after 4-5 weeks, start looking into your dietary choices.

The first thing people typically recommend is re-tracking your macros to make sure you've been on track, making sure you're drinking enough water and supplementing electrolytes, and finally reducing the amount of dairy being used. You can also read more about weight loss plateau's here >

I don't like meat/eggs/dairy, can I still do a ketogenic diet?

A: The short answer is yes. Aside from the broad guidelines stated above, there are no real "rules," so as long as you're low carb, moderate protein and getting the rest of your calories from fat. If it fits within your macros, then you're fine.

Some drink coffee with butter (recipe here) and eat plenty of meat; some do vegetarian recipes, some are dairy and nut free. There are lots of options out there to suit any dietary restriction.

What happens after you reach your goal weight on keto?

A: Some people want to go off keto once they've reached their goal weight, others choose to stay on keto or take up a clean-eating diet. I've been on keto for almost a decade now. One thing to always remember – if you go back to your old habits you will put the weight back on.

If you keep your intake in check, you may still notice an increase in weight because of glycogen stores refilling. Many people find they stick to keto or a low-carb diet simply because it makes them feel better.

Saving Money and Budgeting

Saving money on low-carb

A common misconception is the ketogenic diet is more expensive than other diets out there. And, while it may be a little bit more expensive than buying grain-stuffed foods, it's much cheaper than many people think.

A ketogenic diet may be more expensive than a standard American diet, but it's no different than other clean eating lifestyles. That said, there's still numerous ways to save money while cooking keto. The best ways to save money is the same as with any other budgeting option:

Search for deals. There's always a sale or a coupon to be found for keto-friendly items out there. Typically you can find significant savings in magazines and newspapers that are sent to your house, but they can also be combined with in-store specials and manager cuts. When combined, you can save a significant amount of your keto groceries.

Bulk buys and cooking. If you're someone who doesn't like to spend a lot of time in the kitchen, this is the best of both worlds. Buying your food at bulk (specifically from wholesalers) can reduce the cost per pound tremendously. Plus, you can make ahead food (bulk cook chicken thighs for pre-made meat, or cook entire meals) that are used as leftovers, so you spend less time cooking.

Make things yourself. While it's extremely convenient to buy most things pre-made or pre-cooked, it always adds to the price per pound on items. Try prepping veggies ahead of time instead of buying pre-cut ones. Try making your stew meat from a chuck roast. Or, simply try to make your mayo and salad dressings at home. The simplest of things can work to cut down on your overall grocery shopping.

Takeaways and Advice

Overall, eating a high amount of fat, moderate protein, and low amount of carbs can have a massive impact on your health – lowering your cholesterol, body weight, blood sugar, and raising your energy and mood levels.

A ketogenic diet can be hard to fathom in the beginning, but isn't as hard as it's made out to be. The transition can be a little bit tough, but the growing popularity of the clean eating movement makes it easier and easier to find available low-carb foods.

After reading this page in its entirety, my best cut and dry advice for someone starting off and wanting to lose weight are listed below:

Keep it straightforward and strict. You usually see better results in people who restrict their carb intake further. Try to keep your carbs as low as possible for the first month of keto. Keep it strict by cutting out excess sweets and artificial sweeteners altogether (like diet soda). Cutting these out dramatically decreases sugar cravings.

Drink water and supplement electrolytes. Most common problems come from dehydration or lack of electrolytes. When you start keto (and even in the long run), make sure that you drink plenty of water, salt your foods, and take a multivitamin.

If you're still experiencing issues, you can order electrolyte supplements individually.

Track what you eat. It's so easy to over-consume on carbs when they're hidden in just about everything you pick up. Keeping track of what you eat helps control your carb intake and keep yourself accountable.

HOW TO START THE KETO DIET?

First and foremost, when starting to any diet, you should be committed, because getting in a state of ketosis for sustained periods long enough to enjoy the therapeutic effects of ketones is actually quite a difficult thing to do. It doesn't happen by chance. Being in ketosis does not necessarily mean you are burning fat, or adapted and failure to prepare is preparing to fail.

Here are some basic tips on how to get started:

Getting started is simple: just dive in! It's always good to spend some time cleaning out your kitchen pantry and adding in new staples. Check out our recommendations to start if you're new and not sure what to get. Do a comprehensive research about Keto and decide if the ketogenic diet and lifestyle is right for you.

Visit to a doctor for a full physical examination. Ask them to compute your body fats, weight, height, glucose count calories and body muscles. This will also give you an indication of your starting position.

You can also consult a Keto expert or Keto coach who can give you a comprehensive breakdown of the realities of starting a ketogenic lifestyle and teach you how to compute your macros in order for you to reach the state of ketosis, get through the flu and adaptation. They will also be able to share cost-saving tips for monitoring progress and practical hints for keto meal prep. Sometimes coaches also offer keto meal services developed by nutritionist experts that prepare your meals and deliver it to your home or office.

If you are working on a budget, you can find almost anything and everything you need online from how to calculate macros, meal plans, recipes, meal prep ideas and how to beat the temptation with keto-compliant snacks that you should always have at the ready just in case your mind starts playing tricks on you.

Aim to eat unprocessed whole foods and commit to learning to cook for yourself. It is not just so you know exactly what you are eating, but it is actually mentally rewarding and some careful planning allows you to enjoy your new keto lifestyle without breaking the bank. Make your own food. You will love you for it. We also have a blog which give you tips on keto on a budget. Also, set your carb intake. Normally 20 – 30g per day. The lower the better.

Invest in yourself and your knowledge. Being on keto is often an eye-opener. The first realisation is how much you will feel you have been lied to for most of your life about fats and certain foods. Most people at this point disappear down a rabbit hole for six months and read every clinical study about food facts and fats and carbs, etc. It is not necessary to be Alice in Wonderland. However, it is important to stay ahead and abreast of the latest developments, because going down this route means you are going against the grain and that also puts much of the responsibility for your health on yourself.

Some tools that may be interesting for monitoring progress are a blood glucose monitor and of course the keto strips for testing urine. You can now also get the ketone blood testing strips, but they are very expensive and are not always necessary. For those into high tech, a breath tester can also be acquired for testing ketones in the breath.

Find a community of like-minded people. This is a key success criteria, because many things will happen and it helps not only to have people who have already been through what you are about to go through to guide you, but also people to share delicious meal ideas, and their stories and motivations pictures for inspiration.

Diet is part of a healthy lifestyle and people often forget the rest – such as exercise in boosting mood, well-being reducing saggy skin and you lose weight and building muscle. Exercising helps keep you happy because when you exercise, your body releases chemicals called endorphins.

Drink lots of water. Make it a challenge for yourself to drink a gallon of water every day.

Get that beauty sleep. It does a lot more than keep you beautiful.

Why not give your body a real shot at health, turn a new leaf and stop the bad habits, such as smoking and excessive drinking?

After about three to eight weeks your body will most likely be adapted. Be patient. Your body will reward you.

Be proud and flaunt your achievement.

So, there you have it, I hope you enjoyed reading our ultimate guide for Keto beginners and learned something from us. Stay tuned for our free e-book soon, which is our way of saying thank you for all the love and support you have shown. It will include even more information, more tips for beginners such as meal plans, recipes, meal prep ideas and inspiration, supplements and exercises to get your body and mind in tip top condition.

Ketogenic Weight Loss

How To Use The Ketogenic Diet for Weight Loss

It's pretty obvious the well-known advice to "eat less, move more" for losing weight is not working for most people — if any. In fact, at least ⅔ of dieters who lose weight not only gain it back, but often do so with some extra weight. Yikes. So the question is, can there be a real solution to this problem?

There just might be, and it's a little-known process that more and more people are catching on to: ketosis for weight loss. Ketosis on a low-carb, ketogenic diet works because it helps suppress your appetite unlike other ways of eating. Not only that, it can also support increased focus and mental clarity.

Imagine no longer obsessing about food or worrying about eating too much because your appetite is just… under control. No more counting calories! No more cravings. No more crazy amounts of exercise. Just satiety and a regulated appetite.

Not only that, a ketogenic diet might even be able to help you lose weight faster than other methods — while keeping the weight off. If this idea appeals to you (and come on, how could it not?), you might be ready to try a ketogenic diet for weight loss. But you're still left with some questions, so let's cover all of the details you need to know to get started.

Weight Loss And The Ketogenic Diet

Before you can use a ketogenic diet for weight loss, it's a good idea to have an understanding of how it works. Here are some important points about the ketogenic diet:

A ketogenic diet is centered around bringing the body into a state of ketosis.

Ketosis is metabolic process in which the body burns fat for energy instead of its primary fuel, carbohydrates.

When you drastically cut down on the amount of carbohydrates or calories you're eating, and there aren't enough carbohydrates from food to burn for energy, the body switches to the state of ketosis.

Once in ketosis, the liver uses the body's fatty acids to make molecules known as ketones to burn for fuel. Those on a ketogenic diet eat a low amount of carbs to do just this.

So, why is this good for weight loss? That's what we'll cover next.

Benefits Of Ketosis For Weight Loss

There are many benefits of ketosis for those looking to lose weight on a ketogenic diet, including:

Increased Fat Burn with Ketosis

When you eat low-carb and your body starts burning fat as its primary source of fuel, you're essentially in a fasting state where your body is using your fat stores directly for energy. Those experiencing stalls in their weight loss or having trouble getting rid of unwanted fat can benefit from a ketogenic diet for this reason.

Hormone Regulation with ketosis

Ketosis can help sustain weight loss by regulating hormones that affect weight. After you eat, the hormone cholecystokinin (CCK) is released by your intestines. CCK is responsible for stimulating fat and protein digestion and inhibits the emptying of the stomach, which reduces appetite. This makes CCK a great regulator of food intake. For example, a study in the *American Journal of Clinical Nutrition* showed people injected with CCK stopped eating their meals sooner than those without it.

On the flipside, losing weight can cause your body to secrete less CCK, leading to less satiety after a meal. But this is where ketosis can be helpful. The same study showed that just one week of being in ketosis you are able to raise levels of CCK back to where it was before weight loss! That means eating a ketogenic diet can help you avoid cravings for food all the time after losing weight, reducing the chance of gaining the weight back.

Appetite Suppression with ketosis

Yep, ketogenic low-carb diets may be helpful in reducing appetite by altering the concentrations of hormones and nutrients that affect hunger. It's no wonder ketosis is used as a strategy for weight loss; it removes the need to eat more or respond to cravings for unhealthy foods. This means you can better listen to your body's true hunger signals without worrying about counting calories or going hungry.

Blood Sugar Regulation with ketosis

When you're eating a ketogenic diet full of healthy fats and proteins plus an abundance of vegetables, you experience more stabilized blood sugar. This is much better than traditional diet foods that are usually high in refined sugars and other carbohydrates, leading to a spike in blood sugar that leaves you feeling hungry again soon after.

As you can see, those on a ketogenic diet have an advantage over other forms of weight loss because they increase the chance of maintaining weight loss, reducing cravings, and eliminating the need to stress and obsess over every calorie or food portions.

Weight Loss Benefits In Ketosis

Now the question becomes: how do you use a ketogenic diet for weight loss? And it all starts with reaching ketosis.

How to Reach Ketosis for Weight Loss

Going into ketosis begins with analyzing and shifting your intake of carbohydrates in your diet. On a ketogenic diet, the goal is to limit your carb intake to between 20-50 grams of carbs per day, including those from processed and whole food sources.

A ketogenic diet for weight loss is usually broken down into the following macronutrient percentages:

- High fat intake making up 70-80% of total calories

- Moderate protein intake making up 20-25% of total calories

- Low carb intake making up 5-10% of total calories

These numbers might vary slightly depending on each person and factors like lean body mass, gender, height and weight, and level of activity, but generally they are around the same for most people.

SECTION 2:

KETO BREAD AND LOW CARB

KETO BREAD

The keto diet is the high-fat, moderate-protein, super-low-carb craze you've probably read about online or heard your coworker rave about. And while it has helped countless people lose weight, the rules of what you can and can't eat are pretty restrictive.

In general, you should aim to eat fewer than 50 carbs a day to keep your body in the fat-burning state of ketosis. The general macro breakdown is 70 to 80 percent fat, 15 to 20 percent protein, and five to 10 percent carbs. Since carbs are present in many healthy, keto-friendly foods such as leafy, nonstarchy vegetables and low-sugar fruit, it's generally recommended to stay away from other grains and carb-heavy starches. Yes, this includes bread and all the beloved bread products. Luckily, there's a caveat.

"While traditional bread — yes, even whole wheat and whole grain — is too high in carbohydrates to include on a ketogenic diet, there are several great low-carb bread recipes and products that can be included if you miss the occasional sandwich or roll with your meal," registered dietitian Sarah Koenck, member of the clinical team at Virta Health, told POPSUGAR.

Most bread is made from wheat flours and is one of the most prominent sources of carbohydrates. On average, a slice (28g) of bread provides around 15g of carbohydrates – which is defined as a "one carb serving." However, carbs in bread vary depending on bread type. But not only that, a bread's nutritional profile varies greatly from one loaf to another.

If you're following a keto diet, you're likely interested to know more about carbs in bread and other nutrition facts about bread. Keep reading to learn if and how bread can fit into a low-carb eating plan such as keto.

Types Of Bread

Bread is a type of food made from a dough containing flour and water. Most often, a leavening agent such as yeast and baking soda is used and the dough is baked. There are hundreds of different types of bread made from a variety of grains and through different preparation methods. Below are just a couple of the most well-known examples:

White bread

White bread encompasses a broad category of breads made from milled wheat that has had the outer layers removed, i.e. refined grains. Milled flour does not contain the bran and has a white color. It also has a longer shelf life but not many vitamins, minerals, antioxidants, and no fiber. In the US, white bread is often referred to as sandwich bread. Examples of white breads include plain loaf, ciabatta, and baguette.

Whole wheat bread

Also called wholemeal bread, whole wheat bread is made from flour that contains all parts of the grain, i.e. whole wheat flour. Whole wheat bread has a brown color and is rich in fiber and micronutrients. Examples of whole wheat bread include rye bread, oat bread, and plain whole wheat bread.

Multigrain bread

As the name implies, multigrain bread is bread made from flour of two or more different types of grain. It may include grains such as wheat, barley, millet, and flax. Many multigrain breads also include seeds such as sesame seeds and sunflower seeds. Most multigrain breads are made from whole grain flour, but some may contain a combination of refined grains.

Sourdough bread

Most bread today is leavened with baker's yeast or baking soda. But during early bread-making days, humans made bread using sourdough. Sourdough is made using naturally occurring lactobacilli and yeast in wheat. Sourdough bread has a mildly sour taste and a longer shelf-life than other breads. It also has unique nutritional properties, and there's evidence that it's better for glycemic control than other breads [1].

Sprouted bread

Sprouted bread is made from a special type of flour from germinated grains. Sprouted bread has slightly fewer carbohydrates and more protein than bread from unsprouted grains. Sprouted grains are also easier to digest than unsprouted grains.

How Many Carbs In Bread?

Bread is a significant source of carbohydrates in many countries. Along with rice, it accounts for 40% of the calories consumed worldwide [3]. The exact amount of carbs in a serving of bread (one slice) varies greatly depending on bread type, but the average is estimated around 15g per slice. Below are the exact carb amounts in different types of bread.

- Classic White Bread – 12 grams carbohydrate

- Whole Wheat Bread – 12 grams carbohydrate

- Sprouted Whole Grain Bread – 15 grams carbohydrate

- Brown Rice Bread – 19 grams carbohydrate

- Multigrain Bread – 19 grams carbohydrate

The exact type of carb in these breads also varies. Bread made from refined white flour contains many of the same complex carbs as whole grain bread. However, the lack of fiber in this type of bread means that it is digested quickly, leading to blood sugar spikes. Fiber is an important type of indigestible carbohydrate essential for normal overall health and functioning

How Many Calories In Bread?

The term calorie refers to energy from food. You get all your calories from three macronutrients: protein, fat, and carbohydrates. Carbohydrates and protein provide 4 calories per gram, while fat provides 9 calories per gram. Bread usually contains all three macronutrients in varying amounts. Whole grain bread also contains fiber, which does not provide any calories because your body does not digest it.

With all that taken into account, how many calories are there in bread? As always, it depends on the type. For example, a slice of commercially-prepared whole wheat bread provides around 69 calories. Of these, 66% are coming from digestible carbohydrates, 12% from fat, and 20% from protein.

On the other hand, white bread provides 66 calories per slice, of which 77% is from carbohydrates, 10% from fat, and 10% from protein.

Some breads may also contain ingredients such as milk, butter, eggs, oil, nuts, seeds, and legume flours. This will greatly impact their overall nutritional profile, including calories. Brioche, which is a type of French bread with butter and eggs, provides 150 calories in a slice.

Nutritional Value Of Bread

Bread is an important food staple across the globe. When eaten in its unrefined form, it's a great source of fiber and other nutrients. For example, a thick slice of homemade whole wheat bread provides the following:

- Fiber – 2.8g

- Total fat – 2.5g

- Folate – 29mg

- Niacin – 1.8mg

- Selenium – 17.8mg

- Magnesium – 37.3mg

White bread may also be fortified with important nutrients such as folic acid and iron. Still, most studies show that replacing whole grain bread with white bread reduces your risk of metabolic diseases. Whole grain bread is more satiating due to its higher fiber content and slow digestibility. White bread also provides only empty calories and leads to blood sugar spikes, which is a known cause of overeating and hunger pangs.

Can You Eat Bread On The Keto Diet?

Eating whole grain bread on a well-balanced standard diet is perfectly ok. But on keto, bread is not allowed and defeats the purpose of this diet. The ketogenic diet is a low-carb diet, meaning that it excludes foods that are high in carbohydrates such as bread. But why is this so?

Well, the ketogenic diet is meant to put the body into ketosis, i.e. boost ketone production. The word "ketogenic" means ketone generating. The only way to put the body in a state of ketosis is to reduce carbohydrate intake low enough so the body cannot derive energy from this macronutrient. As a result, it looks for other energy substrates such as fat and produces ketones in the process to help fuel the brain (the brain is one of the rare organs that cannot use fat for fuel).

Because bread provides a significant amount of carbohydrates even at small serving sizes, it is not practical in helping lower carb intake to the recommended 20-50g/day on a ketogenic diet. That's why many keto dieters make bread from non-wheat flours to help lower their daily carb intake (more on that later). Others simply stick to low-carb food such as nuts, seeds, avocados, spinach, and cucumbers.

HEALTH BENEFITS OF BREAD

Carbs in Bread & Other Nutritional Info_infographic_1

While bread is not allowed on keto, but that doesn't mean it's inherently bad. As already explained, whole grain bread is a good source of fiber and nutrients. If eaten alongside a well-planned standard health diet, bread in its whole grain form can contribute to good health. Below are examples of health benefits associated with whole grain bread.

A source of nutrients

Whole wheat bread is a good source of selenium, a trace mineral important for the production of antioxidant enzymes called selenoproteins. Selenium is also essential for reproductive health, thyroid health, and DNA synthesis. Sprouted bread has even greater nutritional value because sprouting removes anti-nutrients, which are compounds that interfere with the absorption of nutrients. Sprouting also increases the number of certain nutrients such as vitamin C, vitamin E, and beta-carotene; however, it's only in negligible amounts.

Reduced disease risk

Public health research shows that consumption of whole wheat bread over refined sources of carbohydrates reduces the risk of several diseases and health outcomes, including:

- Cardiovascular disease: 25%

- Hypertension: 21%

- Digestive tumors: 22%

- Death following a heart attack: 31%

This is likely due to higher fiber intake with whole grain bread as well as the added antioxidants found in unrefined grains. For example, fiber feeds god gut bacteria, which produce short-chain fatty acids like butyric acid when fermenting fiber. Studies show butyric acid protects the health of gut tissue.

Greater satiety

Hunger and satiety play an important role in weight management. These responses to food intake depend a lot on blood glucose levels and your overall metabolic health. Blood sugar spikes caused by intake of refined carbohydrates, for instance, lead to greater insulin release and subsequent blood sugar drops that cause strong feelings of hunger shortly thereafter [10].

You can prevent this by switching to whole grain bread. Whole grain bread contains more fiber, which helps slow down the breakdown of starch in the bread. This leads to a gradual release in blood glucose. Fiber also creates bulk in the digestive system, and this also seems to contribute to greater satiety. However, switching to a low-carb diet is your best option when it comes to appetite control according to studies [11].

How To Eat Bread On Keto?

Eating bread on a standard keto diet is not allowed. However, you can eat bread on a cyclical ketogenic diet (CKD) and on the targeted ketogenic diet (TKD). Both versions of keto allow for occasional carb refeeding to help replenish glycogen stores. Here is how that works:

CKD

The CKD involves 5-6 days of standard ketogenic eating, i.e. restricting carbs to fewer than 50g a day. This is then followed by 1-2 days of eating up to 150g of carbohydrates a day. This helps replenish glycogen stores in the muscles and liver. It also kicks you out of ketosis temporarily. The proposed benefits of the CKD over the standard ketogenic diet include better workouts, greater muscle recovery and growth, and improved thyroid functioning.

TKD

On a TKD, you eat more carbs only around your workouts. This is best suitable for highly athletic folk. Like the CKD, the TKD also helps replenish muscle glycogen, which is important for muscle recovery following rigorous workouts. However, it isn't really necessary as new studies show you can get just as many benefits through keto-adaptation, which requires at least 6 weeks of being on a standard keto diet .

In both cases, the source of carbs doesn't matter, so you can feel free to even eat white bread to replenish your glycogen stores. In fact, white bread may even be a better option on a TKD since it's easier to digest and turn to glucose and glycogen.

However, if you want to follow a standard keto diet, then you should consider low-carb bread alternatives. These are often referred to as keto breads. Keto breads are simply breads made from nut flours such as almond flour, hazelnut flour, and coconut flour. The most popular flour to make keto breads is almond flour.

Because almond flour is high in fat, low in carbs, and does not contain gluten, it behaves differently than wheat flour during baking. Using yeast won't work with almond flour, so you should use baking powder and eggs instead. Another low-carb alternative to wheat bread is cloud bread, an egg-based bread with cream of tartar.

How to make the best keto bread

When preparing keto bread recipes, look out for low-carb ingredients that could contribute to brain fog and inflammation. Skip recipes that require conventional dairy or yeast, and avoid eating common keto bread ingredients like psyllium husk, xanthan gum, and nuts or nut butters too often — these can contain mold or irritate your gut. Grass-fed butter, ghee, and coconut flour are the few exceptions that will still produce a stellar loaf.

Takeaways

Bread is an important food staple across the globe.

There are hundreds of different bread varieties; however, several types of wheat bread are among the most commonly consumed and include white bread, whole grain bread, sourdough bread, rye bread, and sprouted grain bread.

Bread is normally not allowed on keto because it contains too many carbohydrates to make it practical on this low-carb diet.

The only time you can eat bread on keto is if you're following a cyclical or targeted keto diet.

There are some low-carb breads made using nut flours and eggs that have a similar taste, shape, and texture as wheat bread.

WHAT IS LOW CARB?

What is a low carb diet? Well, it doesn't take a scientific mind to realize people, and Americans especially, have difficulty choosing the right foods and an adequate quantity of those foods. To put it lightly, our diets are awful. We are obese with elevated cholesterol levels and blood pressure, and are crippled by arthritis and cancer. Although many maladies are dependent on one's genetic makeup and can hardly be avoided, a lot can be said for eating wholesome foods to help fortify your body.

The Basics

Eat: Meat, fish, eggs, vegetables growing above ground and natural fats (like butter).

Avoid: Sugar and starchy foods (like bread, pasta, rice, beans and potatoes).

Eat when you're hungry, until you're satisfied. It can be that simple. You do not need to count calories or weigh your food. And just forget about industrially produced low-fat products

Many people with diabetes are following a low-carb diet because of its benefits in terms of improving diabetes control, weight loss and being a diet that is satisfying and easy to stick to.

Low-carb diets are flexible and can be followed by people with different types of diabetes.

The diet has allowed many people with type 2 diabetes to resolve their diabetes, that is to get their blood sugar levels into a non-diabetic range without the help of medication.

People with type 1 diabetes have also reported much more stable blood sugar levels, making the condition easier to predict and manage.

The diet is a healthy way of eating as vegetables and natural, real foods are integral to the diet.

One of the most popular diets on the market these days are the low carb diets, such as Atkins, South Beach, or the Zone. Low carb diets typically advocate portion control and a concept called insulin control. When one eats a highly refined, sugary Twinkie, the bloodstream is inundated with glucose within 7 minutes and not too much later, the pancreas releases excessive amounts of insulin to transport the blood glucose to where it needs to go. This causes your blood sugar levels to plummet and for the excess glucose to be stored as fat. This, of course, leads to obesity and heart disease.

So, instead of eating processed, sugary foods, one needs to eat what are called "complex carbohydrates." These cause a more gradual climb in blood sugar levels and therefore provide more energy that lasts longer. This ingrained pattern of eating junk food out of laziness is what the low carb diets are trying to get rid of.

Instead, they are advocating an restriction on starchy pastas, potatoes, and breads, while advocating an increased consumption of good protein sources and fresh vegetables and fruits. According to research, by ingesting more protein, one's metabolism has to work harder to break it down for use as energy, thus raising the metabolic rate.

So, not only will you be burning more calories, but by limiting the intake of starchy carbs, one is protecting themselves from the complications of type II diabetes. So, low carb, high protein diets seem to make sense but is there scientific merit to their claims?

Yes, when one lowers their intake of starchier and more refined carbs, there are numerous health benefits that come with the territory. First of all, research has proven people can lose substantial weight on a low carb diet without restricting calories.

Low carb, high protein diets can help lower triglyceride levels, increase HDL cholesterol levels, reduce blood glucose levels for diabetics as well as non-diabtetics, improve insulin sensitivity, lower blood pressure, improve concentration due to regulated blood glucose levels, and lower blood insulin levels.

Others have made unsubstantiated claims that low carb, high protein diets left them with fewer headaches, lessened PMS symptoms, healthier looking skin, and even better joint motion.

One thing you should understand is there are essentially two kinds of carbs. They are simple and complex carbs. In most cases, the former will be regarded as bad carbs. And without any surprise, the latter are usually regarded as good carbohydrates.

When simple carbohydrates are concerned, the fact here is that they can be digested quickly. These will of course lead to an increase of blood glucose level. Because of the rise in glucose level, your body will produce more insulin. And of course the result is you will gain fat a lot easier. You can get simple carbohydrates easily from foods such as white bread and soda.

On the other hand, complex carbs are something different. In most cases, foods with high fiber contents contains complex carbohydrates. The point here is they are usually healthier. As a result, there should be no harm for you to eat such carbohydrates. In most cases, whole grains and vegetables will contain complex carbs.

So, if you are considering trying a low carb diet, it is important that you try to cut the consumption of foods which contain simple carbohydrates. On the other hand, you should try to consume some good carbohydrates. This will certainly help you to lose weight. In fact, studies have already shown you can lose weight effectively with such a diet plan!

Of course it will be quite difficult for us to cut all the consumption of simple carbohydrates. The idea here is you should avoid them as much as you can. The baseline here is that you should at least avoid soda and other sugary foods. If you can take this kind of healthy low carb diet, you will be able to lose weight eventually!

How do low-carb diets work? They're effective because they cause glucose to quickly run out, and when your supply becomes low enough, your body turns to fat for fuel as a backup source — whether it's fat coming from your diet, or your own stored body fat.

Our bodies normally run on glucose or sugar for energy, but we cannot make glucose ourselves and only store about 24 hours worth within our muscles and liver. Once glucose from carbohydrates is no longer available for energy due to following a low-carb diet, we begin to burn stored fat for fuel instead. This is why low-carb diets often lead to fast weight loss and other metabolic improvements within a relatively short period of time.

THE DIFFERENCE BETWEEN LOW-CARB DIETS: HIGH-FAT VS. HIGH-PROTEIN

People can mean different things when referring to low-carb diets, which creates some confusion about what a low-carb diet might actually look like. For example, which type of low-carb diet is more common and more beneficial, high-fat or high-protein?

High-Fat, Low-Carb Diets (aka the Ketogenic Diet):

A ketogenic diet — one form of a very low-carb diet — is a high-fat diet that strictly eliminates almost all sources of glucose in order to put the body into "fat-burning mode," also called nutritional ketosis. The ketogenic diet goes by several different names, including the "no-carb diet" or "very low carbohydrate ketogenic diet"(LCKD or VLCKD for short).

Ketogenic diets have been used by doctors to treat patients with epilepsy and metabolic conditions since the 1920s! They have well-documented benefits, including helping to treat epilepsy, promoting rapid weight loss and reducing diabetes risk. Not only have studies over the past century shown that the keto diet can reduce the amount of seizures patients suffer from, but it can also have positive effects on body fat, blood sugar, cholesterol levels, hunger levels and neurological health. (1)

When you're following a traditional ketogenic diet, you consume about about 75 percent of your daily calories from healthy fats, just about 5 percent from carbohydrates, and about 20 percent from protein.

Ketogenic diets limit daily net carb intake to just 20–30 grams (net carbs are the amount of carb leftover when fiber is subtracted from total carbs).

While the keto diet is a great fit for the right type of person, many people will still experience great results when eating a modified keto diet that is a bit higher in carbs, or "keto-cycling" or "carb-cycling" in which they boost carb intake on certain days of the week.

Compared to high-protein diets, the ketogenic diet is considered "moderate protein." It's important not to over-consume protein on the keto diet because this can interfere with your ability to produce ketone bodies for energy and to enter nutritional ketosis.

You might have concern over how restrictive a ketogenic diet will be, and maybe you're concerned about side effects or "carb withdrawal." Initially, keto diets can cause some side effects that typically last 1–2 weeks.

However, data from certain clinical trials has shown that low-carb diets, even very low-carb ketogenic diets, can actually help improve mood and reduce fatigue and hunger. A 2007 study conducted by the Department of Psychiatry and Behavioral Sciences at Duke University Medical Center found that participants experienced significant improvements in a broad range of negative symptoms when following a very low-carb diet, even more so than participants following a low-fat diet. Those on the very low-carb reported less fatigue, cognitive symptoms, physical effects of hunger, insomnia and stomach problems than the low-fat diet group. (4)

High-Protein, Low-Carb Diets:

Generally speaking, people who are not intentionally controlling their protein take usually get about 15–25 percent of their daily calories from protein foods.

If you choose to follow a high-protein diet, your diet will be roughly distributed as 30 to 35 percent protein, 20 percent or less carbohydrates, and about 45 to 50 percent fat. With every meal you'll want to incorporate 1–2 palm-sized portions of protein, such as fish or meat. (3)

The main difference between high-fat and high-protein diets is the amount of protein — in the form of meat, fish, eggs, etc. — that someone is eating. Higher-fat diets like the keto diet call for more healthy fats in the form of butter, oil and fattier cuts of meat, while higher-protein diets still include fats, but less.

WHAT CAN YOU EAT ON A LOW-CARB DIET?

How many carbs should you eat in a day on a low-carb diet? Depending on who you ask, a low-carbohydrate diet can include any diet that involves getting less than 30 to 40 percent of daily calories/energy from carbohydrates.

Forty percent of your diet consisting of carbs is still a relatively high amount, so if you're aiming to eat low-carb, you'll probably want to consume a good deal less than this. On the other hand, low-fat diets are those that involve getting 25 to 30 percent or less of daily calories/energy from fat.

Each person is different, but generally reducing carbohydrates to about 30 percent of your overall diet, while increasing fat to 40 percent and protein to 30 percent, is a great target to aim for.

From there, you might choose to further tweak your macronutrient intake ("macronutrients" are fats, carbs and protein) to reach certain goals, for example, entering ketosis via a ketogenic diet.

So, how many carbs are included in a low carb diet? If you eat 2,000 to 2,500 calories per day, getting 30 percent of your daily calories from carbs would equate to about 150 grams to 187 grams of carbs per day (each gram of carbs contains roughly 4 calories).

You can consider this amount to be relatively low-carb, although it's still a much higher carb intake then you'd eat on a diet like the ketogenic diet.

The best way to start eating a lower-carb diet is to simply focus on eliminating major sources of added sugar and carbohydrates — especially from sugar snacks, sweetened drinks, grains and possibly legumes and dairy, too. At the same time, work on increasing calories from healthy fats and quality proteins. By following these guidelines, most adults will see fast weight loss and improvements in overall health.

Keep in mind everyone reacts differently to various dietary plans, and there isn't necessarily a one-size-fits-all approach to low-carb dieting that is going to work best for everyone. Factors like someone's age, gender, level of activity, bodyweight and genetic disposition all affect how that person feels when following a low-carb diet.

Therefore, it's important to practice self-awareness if you plan to reduce your carb intake in order to arrive at the level of carbs in your diet that works best for you personally. This might take some trial and error initially, and it's usually best to reduce carbs gradually in order to prevent side effects like cravings or being tired.

1. Healthy Fats

Most healthy fats contain zero net carbs, especially the kinds listed below, which also have other health advantages. (4) Fats should be included in high amounts with every meal throughout the day.

Healthy fats include saturated fats, monounsaturated fats and certain types of polyunsaturated fats (PUFAs), especially omega-3 fatty acids. It's best to include all types in your diet, with an emphasis on saturated fats, especially compared to PUFAs.

MCT oil, cold-pressed coconut, palm fruit, olive oil, flaxseed, macadamia and avocado oil, butter and ghee, avocado, lard, chicken fat or duck fat are all good choices.

2. Quality Proteins

Animal proteins (meat, fish, etc.) have very little, if any, carbs. You can consume them in moderate amounts as needed to control hunger. Overall, choose organic, grass-fed and fattier cuts of meat rather than leaner ones. For example, chicken thighs and legs are preferable to chicken breasts because they contain much more fat.

Grass-fed beef and other types of fatty cuts of meat, including lamb, goat, veal, venison and other game. Grass-fed, fatty meat is preferable because it's higher in quality omega-3 fats.

Organ meats including liver

Poultry, including turkey, chicken, quail, pheasant, hen, goose, duck

Cage-free eggs and egg yolks

Fish, including tuna, trout, anchovies, bass, flounder, mackerel, salmon, sardines, etc.

3. Non-Starchy Vegetables

All leafy greens, including dandelion or beet greens, collards, mustard, turnip, arugula, chicory, endive, escarole, fennel, radicchio, romaine, sorrel, spinach, kale, chard, etc.

Cruciferous veggies like broccoli, cabbage, Brussels sprouts and cauliflower

Celery, cucumber, zucchini, chives and leeks

Fresh herbs

Veggies that are slightly higher in carbs (but still low all things considered) include asparagus, mushrooms, bamboo shoots, bean sprouts, bell pepper, sugar snap peas, water chestnuts, radishes, jicama, green beans, wax beans, tomatoes

Avocado (technically a fruit)

4. Full-Fat Dairy

Dairy products should be limited to only "now and then" due to containing natural sugars. Higher fat, hard cheeses have the least carbs, while low-fat milk and soft cheeses have much more.

Full-fat cow's and goat milk (ideally organic and raw) and full-fat cheeses.

5. Snacks

Bone broth (homemade or protein powder)

Beef or turkey jerky

Hard-boiled eggs

Extra veggies (raw or cooked) with homemade dressing

1/2 avocado with sliced lox (salmon)

Minced meat wrapped in lettuce

6. Condiments

Spices and herbs, hot sauce, apple cider vinegar, unsweetened mustards, cocoa, powder, vanilla extract, and stevia

7. Drinks

Water, unsweetened coffee (black) and tea, fresh made vegetable juice, and bone broth

Foods to Eat in Limited Amounts

You'll want to limit foods including medium-starchy veggies that contain more carbs (like sweet peas, artichokes, okra, carrots, beets and parsnips, yams and potatoes), legumes, beans, fruit and dairy products like yogurt/kefir.

The amount you have of these will depend on how low-carb of a diet you're following. As a general rule, have no more than 1/2 cup serving cooked per day.

What Should You Not Eat on a Low-Carb Diet?

1. Any Type of Sugar

White, brown, cane, raw and confectioner's sugar

Syrups like maple, carob, corn, caramel and fruit

Honey and agave

Any food made with ingredients such as fructose, glucose, maltose, dextrose and lactose

2. Any and All Grains

One slice of bread, or small serving of grains, can have anywhere from 10–30 net grams of carbs! Cereals and cooked grains typically have 15–35 grams per 1/4 cup uncooked, depending on the kind.

Wheat, oats, all rice (white, brown, jasmine), quinoa, couscous, pilaf, etc.

Corn and all products containing corn, including popcorn, tortillas, grits, polenta and cornmeal

All types of products made with flour, including bread, bagels, rolls, muffins, pasta, etc.

3. Nearly All Processed Foods

Crackers, chips, pretzels, etc.

All types of candy

All desserts like cookies, cakes, pies, ice cream

Pancakes, waffles and other baked breakfast items

Oatmeal and cereals

Snack carbs, granola bars, most protein bars or meal replacements, etc.

Canned soups, boxed foods, any prepackaged meal

Foods containing artificial ingredients like artificial sweeteners (sucralose, aspartame, etc.), dyes and flavors

4. Sweetened and Caloric Beverages

Soda

Alcohol (beer, wine, liquor, etc.)

Sweetened teas or coffee drinks

Milk and dairy replacements (cow's milk, soy, almond, coconut, Lactaid®, cream, half and half, etc.)

Fruit juices

Can you eat fruit on a low-carb diet? If so, which fruit has the least carbs? Berries, including blueberries, strawberries, blackberries, raspberries, are the best choice because they are nutrient-dense and low in carbs. Stick to about 1/4 to 1/2 cup per day.

8 BENEFITS OF A LOW-CARB DIET

1. Fast Weight Loss

When it comes to losing weight, calorie counting is crazy, but shifting your attention to the types of foods you eat and focusing on mindful eating can make all the difference. Low-carb diets have a reputation for producing fast weight loss without feeling hungry or needing to count calories. In fact, many people experience weight loss following a low-carb diet even if they've tried "everything else" and never got the results they were looking for.

A 2014 study conducted by the National Institutes of Health found that after comparing the two in overweight adults, low-carb diets were more effective for weight loss and cardiovascular risk factor reduction compared to low-fat diets, as demonstrated by 148 participants following both types of dietary plans over 12 months.

Why are low-carb diets, especially the keto diet, so effective for shedding excess pounds, even in people who normally struggle to lose weight? When we eat foods with sugar and carbohydrates, the hormone insulin is released as a reaction in order to elevate blood glucose (sugar). Insulin is often called a "fat-storage hormone" because one of its jobs is to signal cells to store as much available energy as possible. This energy is initially stored as glycogen from the glucose found in carbohydrates, since glycogen is our "primary" energy.

By eliminating carbohydrates from the diet and keeping the body's glycogen stores low or almost empty, we can prevent insulin from being released and storing fat. Less insulin circulating around our bloodstream means that the body is forced to use up all of its glycogen stores, then reach into fat stores tucked away in our adipose tissue (body fat) for ongoing fuel.

2. Better Cognitive Function

Fat and carbohydrates usually have an inverse relationship in someone's diet. Most people keep protein intake somewhat steady, but normally the more carbs and sugar people eat, the less healthy fats they consume. This is problematic because we need healthy fats for proper brain function, mood control and hormone regulation. While initially a sugary or high-carb meal might make you feel awake and alert, quickly after you'll likely come crashing down and might feel tired, grumpy and irritable.

Sugar is addictive and has dramatic effects on the brain, especially when it comes to increasing cravings, anxiety and fatigue. On the other hand, certain kinds of healthy fats, including cholesterol, act like antioxidants and precursors to some important brain-supporting molecules and neurotransmitters that control learning, memory, mood and energy. Your brain is largely made up of fatty acids and requires a steady stream of fats from your diet in order to perform optimally.

Recently, a 2012 report published in The Journal of Physiology found evidence of strong metabolic consequences of a high-sugar diet coupled with a deficiency of omega-3 fatty acids on cognitive abilities. These effects were due to the association of consuming high amounts of glucose and insulin action, which control brain-signaling mediators. As one might expect, the unhealthy diet that was high in sugar but low in healthy fats like omega-3 fatty acids was associated with lower cognitive scores and insulin resistance.

Research suggests the ketogenic diet is especially therapeutic when it comes to protecting cognitive health. Researchers believe that people with the highest insulin resistance might demonstrate a lower cerebral blood flow and, therefore, less brain plasticity.

This is because insulin is a "vasodilator" and increases blood flow to promote glucose delivery to the muscles and organs, including the brain. This vasodilator function is stopped when someone develops insulin resistance over time from a high-sugar and high-carb intake, resulting in a decrease in perfusion of brain tissues and activity.

In certain studies, improvement have been observed in Alzheimer's disease and dementia patients fed a ketogenic diet, marked by factors including improved mitochondrial function. A European *Journal of Clinical Nutrition* study pointed to emerging data that suggested the therapeutic use of ketogenic diets for multiple neurological disorders beyond epilepsy and Alzheimer's, including headaches, neurotrauma, Parkinson's disease, sleep disorders, brain cancer, autism and multiple sclerosis.

3. Reduced Risk of Metabolic Syndrome and Heart Disease

A 2012 study published in *The American Journal of Epidemiology* found that low-carbohydrate diets are more effective at reducing certain metabolic and heart disease risk factors than low-fat diets are, plus at least equally effective at reducing weight and other factors.

The study investigated the effects of low-carbohydrate diets (≤45 percent of energy from carbohydrates) versus low-fat diets (≤30 percent of energy from fat) on metabolic risk factors by conducting a meta-analysis of randomized controlled trials. Twenty-three trials from multiple countries with a total of 2,788 participants were included in the analyses.

The results showed both low-carbohydrate and low-fat diets lowered weight and improved metabolic risk factors. But compared with participants on low-fat diets, people on low-carbohydrate diets experienced a significantly greater increase in "good" high-density lipoprotein cholesterol and a greater decrease in triglycerides.

They also experienced a lower reduction in total cholesterol and low-density lipoprotein cholesterol than the low-fat diet group. However, keep in mind that higher cholesterol levels have not been proven to contribute to heart disease!

These findings were true despite the fact that reductions in body weight, waist circumference and other metabolic risk factors were not significantly different between the two diet groups. These findings suggest that satisfying lower-carb diets, which are higher in fat, can help beat heart disease factors just as well as diets that are harder to stick with and are prone to leaving people hungry.

4. Lower Risk for Type-2 Diabetes

Researchers point out that despite the growing rates of type 1 and 2 diabetes and the accelerating cost of the resources needed to monitor and treat diabetic patients, the medical community generally hasn't been successful at reducing either the number of people affected or the severity of the complications. While prescriptions for diabetes medications continue to climb, there's a simple, effective, low-cost strategy that is proven to work with diabetes: Reduce the amount of sugar and starch in the diet.

Researchers from the Division of Endocrinology, Diabetes and Hypertension at SUNY University of Brooklyn point out that a high-carbohydrate diet raises postprandial plasma glucose and insulin secretion, thereby increasing risk of diabetes, heart disease, hypertension, dyslipidemia and obesity.

Many studies have shown a low-carb diet is a natural diabetes treatment and effective tool in the prevention of patients with type 2 diabetes. It can also help lower risks for diabetes complications and related risk factors like obesity or heart disease.

A growing body of evidence shows that although a diet high in "healthy carbs" like whole grains is still recommended to many sick patients, low-carbohydrate diets are comparable if not better than traditional low-fat/high-carbohydrate diets for weight reduction, improvement in the dyslipidemia of diabetes and metabolic syndrome as well as control of blood pressure, postprandial glycemia and insulin secretion.

In a 2005 study published in *The Upsala Journal of Medical Science*, for two groups of obese patients with type 2 diabetes, the effects of two different diet compositions were tested with regard to glycemic control and body weight. A group of 16 obese patients with type 2 diabetes was put on a low-carb diet (1,800 calories for men and 1,600 calories for women) that consisted of 20 percent carbohydrates, 30 percent protein and 50 percent fat.

Fifteen obese diabetes patients were put on a high-carbohydrate diet to serve as the control group. Their diet consisting of the same calories for men and women included approximately 60 percent carbohydrates, 15 percent protein and 25 percent fat. Positive effects on the glucose levels were seen very quickly in the group following the low-carb plan. After six months, a marked reduction in body weight of patients in the low-carb diet group was also observed, and this remained one year later.

5. Help Fighting Cancer

Research shows that a diet high in refined carbohydrates and sugar contributes to free radical damage and actually feeds cancer cells, possibly helping them proliferate faster. Because low-carb diets dramatically cut down sugar and lower intake of grains and processed foods, they might act like a natural cancer treatment, causing immunity to improve as oxidative stress goes down.

Studies indicate that carbohydrate intake influences prostate cancer biology, as demonstrated through mice that have been fed a no-carbohydrate ketogenic diet (NCKD) experiencing significantly smaller tumors and longer survival times than mice fed a Western diet. The mice fed the equivalent of the standard human Western diet had higher serum insulin, which was associated with significantly higher blood glucose and tumor tissue growth.

In the process of cutting off the supply of energy to cancers, healthy cells are luckily preserved since they're able to use fat for energy. Cancer cells, on the other hand, thrive off of glucose and cannot metabolically shift to use fat.

6. Fewer Cravings and Not Going Hungry!

One of the biggest benefits of a low-carb diet or the keto diet is that eating more healthy fats and proteins in place of sugar and carbohydrates is super satisfying, since it effectively helps turn off ghrelin, the "hungry hormone."

According to studies, insulin negatively regulates ghrelin, and high-density lipoprotein may be a carrier particle for increasing circulating ghrelin. In other words, carbs spike insulin quickly, which leads to cravings for more food later on as blood sugar drops and ghrelin increases. Fats and proteins, on the other hand, are known for switching on the body's satiety hormones and allowing you to go longer comfortably between meals without needing to snack.

According to a report published in *The Journal of International Studies of Obesity*:

Leptin and ghrelin are two hormones that have been recognized to have a major influence on energy balance. Leptin is a mediator of long-term regulation of energy balance, suppressing food intake and thereby inducing weight loss.

Ghrelin on the other hand is a fast-acting hormone, seemingly playing a role in meal initiation. As a growing number of people suffer from obesity, understanding the mechanisms by which various hormones and neurotransmitters have influence on energy balance has been a subject of intensive research. It is now established that obese patients are leptin-resistant.

To get off the roller-coaster of insulin highs and lows, you need to gain control over your primary appetite hormones. The easier way to do this is to keep appetite-boosting sugar low and include quality proteins and fats with every meal, especially in the morning with breakfast, which sets the tone for the entire day.

Ketones that are created by the body during the ketogenic diet have also been shown to help curb hunger and to make intermittent fasting easier. In studies conducted on average weight adults, consumption of ketone supplements has been shown to lead to suppression of ghrelin, reduced hunger and less desire to eat.

7. Better Digestion

Less sugar means better digestive function for most people, since sugar feeds "bad bacteria" that can thrive in the gut. The result of a diet too high in sugar and carbs can mean the development of candida virus, IBS and worsened symptoms of leaky gut syndrome. Plenty of vegetables, quality proteins and healthy fats, on the other hand, can act like fat-burning foods that also help nourish the digestive tract and reduce bacterial growth.

Research from a 2008 study published in the *Journal of the American Gastroenterological Association* showed that patients with irritable bowel syndrome (IBS) report symptom improvements after initiating a very low-carbohydrate diet (VLCD). When participants with moderate to severe IBS were provided a two-week standard diet, then four weeks of a VLCD (20 grams of carbohydrates a day), the majority reported improvements in abdominal pain, stool habits and quality of life.

8. Better Hormone Regulation

You've already learned about the positive effects that a low-carb diet can have on insulin and appetite hormones, but going low-carb appears to also help balance neurotransmitter function in some people and thus improve mood.

When researchers from the Discipline of Psychiatry and School of Medicine at the University of Adelaide compared the hormonal and psychological effects of a low-protein, high-carbohydrate (LPHC) diet and a high-protein, low-carbohydrate (HPLC) diet in women with a hormonal disorder called polycystic ovary syndrome (PCOS) over the course of 16 weeks, they found a significant reduction in depression and improvement in self-esteem in those on the low-carb diet.

All participants attended a weekly exercise, group support and educational program and completed the Hospital Anxiety and Depression Scale at the beginning and end of the study. The HPLC diet appeared to help balance hormones naturally and was associated with significant reductions in various depressive symptoms, enhanced feelings of well-being and higher likelihood of having better compliance with long-term treatment of obesity.

Precautions and Side Effects When Starting a Low-Carb Diet

Overall, there seems to be a lot of variability when it comes to how low-carb dieting and changes in moods and energy levels — with some people feeling great and others struggling a bit initially. This is why it's important to pay attention to how you feel as you change your diet, and make adjustments as necessary.

Self-reports, along with data from certain trials, indicate that very low-carb diets or ketogenic diets might increase symptoms like fatigue, constipation, brain-fog and irritability in some people — side effects that have been nicknamed "the carb flu" or "keto flu." However, this is usually the case when cutting back carbs dramatically to just about 5 percent to 10 percent of total calories. These side effects usually clear up within 1–2 weeks of changing your diet, after your body adjusts.

Obviously, reductions in the desire to be physical active, experiencing brain fog and being cranky are pretty counterproductive for people looking to feel healthier and lose weight, so these effects are something to monitor yourself for. If you're feeling very sluggish, moody, or like you have "brain fog" and can't think clearly while after drastically reducing your carbs over the course of several weeks — especially if you changed your diet rapidly and reduced carbs to very low ketogenic levels — try reintroducing some carbs several days a week until you feel better. Experiencing the benefits of low-carb diets can take some trial and error, plus some patience.

Final Thoughts on Low-Carb Diets:

A low-carb diet is a diet that limits carbohydrates — such as from foods with added sugar, grains, starchy vegetables and fruit — and emphasizes foods high in protein and fat.

Benefits of low-carb diets include: help with weight loss, reduced hunger, better control over insulin and blood sugar, enhanced cognitive performance, lower risk for heart disease factors, improved neurological health, and reduced risk for certain types of cancer.

Low-carb diets tend to be either very high in fat or high in protein. A very high-fat, low-carb diet is called the ketogenic diet. This diet causes the body to create ketones and burn fat for fuel, which has many benefits.

On most low-carb diets, you get about 30 percent or less of daily calories from carbs. Keto diets involve getting 75 percent or more of calories from fat, while high-protein diets usually entail getting 30 percent or more of calories from protein.

Low-carb diets or ketogenic diets might increase symptoms like fatigue, constipation, brain fog and irritability in some people. These side effects usually clear up within 1–2 weeks, although some people will ultimately feel better eating a more moderate-carb diet.

IS LOW-CARB BREAD BETTER FOR YOU THAN REGULAR BREAD?

Low-carb bread is popping up in grocery stores and food blogs everywhere. Whether you're making a quesadilla with a low-carbohydrate tortilla from Whole Foods or trying the Pinterest-famous cloud bread recipe (which is basically a high-protein, carb-free bread popular amongst paleo and keto dieters), the idea of enjoying bread for only half the carbs is certainly intriguing. So we talked to experts to get the full lowdown on the trend.

What is low-carb bread?

"Low-carb breads are similar to gluten-free breads, in that they substitute wheat for something that is lower in carbs," explains Natalie Rizzo, R.D. While the term "low-carb" isn't regulated, meaning that there isn't a universal standard of what makes something low in carbohydrates, she says a piece of low-carb bread typically has half of what you'd get in a piece of regular bread.

"Typically one regular slice of bread has 15 grams of carbs—so if you're having a sandwich that would be 30 grams," says Keri Gans, R.D.N, C.D.N. "Honestly NOT a lot. But if you are following a low-carb diet that may suggest no more than 100 grams total for the day—30 grams might seem like a lot," she says.

What is it made of?

With the rising popularity of paleo and keto diets, many low-carb breads are being made with almond and coconut flours, explains Rizzo. "It could be some other more processed ingredients, like whey protein isolate or soy products," she says. However, when you use other types of flour, you usually need to add more ingredients to make the bread taste like wheat bread, and that's where things can get a little iffy. "Some varieties have a clean ingredient label and are perfectly healthy, but some varieties that include high-fructose corn syrup or tons of weird additives," could be harmful, she says.

Is low-carb bread good for you?

It's not so much that it's bad for you, but low-carb bread alternatives don't have the same nutritional profile as other bread, says Rizzo. "It lacks the whole grains that contain protein and fiber. For instance, a slice of Dave's Killer Bread 21 Whole Grains and Seeds has 22 grams of carbs, five grams of protein, and five grams of fiber, whereas some of the lower-carb options are made with almond and coconut flours that aren't as high in protein and fiber," says Rizzo.

And, when you're skimping on nutrition, especially fiber, you're going to feel less full, so you might get some cravings or a surge in appetite later on, says Gans. "I have found that most patients who eat low-calorie breads wind up being hungrier after lunch than if they had eaten regular 100 percent whole-grain bread," she says.

Should you try it?

"If someone has diabetes, a low-carb bread can help prevent blood sugar spikes," says Rizzo. However, "many people who don't have any health concerns think that low-carb means less calories, but that's not necessarily the case. It's a matter of personal preference, but I don't believe there's any need to try the low-carb varieties of bread," she explains. (Besides, here are a few ways to lose weight without going low-carb.)

SECTION 3:

KETO BREAD RECIPES

KETO BREAD RECIPES

Before I finally took the plunge and went keto a couple of months ago, I wrestled with a serious question: Could I handle life without the occasional sandwich? While the wildly popular high-fat/moderate-protein/restricted-carb diet does allow for certain indulgences — hello, cheese! — I knew that on keto, a lot of my favorite foods were going to be strictly verboten. And that meant waving goodbye to pizza, pasta and my beloved bread.

In an attempt to keep some semblance of sandwich-y goodness in my life, at first I turned to the lettuce wrap. And while some of these quasi-sandwiches were legit delicious — egg salad with olives is a standout — I needed more than that. Because the fact is, when you get hit with a serious craving for bread, a lettuce wrap is just not going to cut it.

The words "keto" and "bread" may seem diametrically opposed—but alas, your desperate, carb-starved self still Googled them together in hopes of a culinary miracle. And we don't blame you one bit. After all, this low-carb, high-fat, moderate-protein keto diet isn't without its grueling transition period known as the keto flu, which can include some pretty intense cravings.

The good news: Even though the keto diet is high in good fats—like avocados and coconut oil—and very low in sugar and carbs, you can definitely still find comfort in your favorite carby flavors and textures without sabotaging your goals. It's all about making strategic ingredient swaps and adding in the appropriate keto-friendly foods.

The ingredients: What makes a bread recipe keto-friendly?

To keep your total carb intake low (so you can stay in that fat-burning state known as ketosis), the best keto bread recipes forgo traditional flour for high-fiber and high-fat ingredients like almond flour, coconut flour, psyllium husk powder, eggs, and healthy fats like grass-fed butter or avocado oil. This not only helps you hit your keto macros, but it ups your intake of some awesome nutrients as well.

Almond flour is packed with vitamin E and magnesium, coconut flour and psyllium husk (which is an amazing binder) are sky-high in fiber to keep blood sugar balanced and boost the health of your microbiome, and glorious eggs are a potent source of choline, vitamin K2, and biotin, among other nutrients.

Together, these ingredients somehow manage to achieve almost-authentic bread flavor. Of course, you're not going to achieve that perfect crumb and bouncy texture of breads made with traditional flour (gluten is responsible for that classic elasticity), but the final product is certainly good enough for your next round of avocado toast.

Subsequently, we are going to talk about 30 friendly and healthy keto bread recipe. so, sit tight and let get started to the main point of the book.

Now, enough with the chit chat. Let's make some keto bread!

BASIC KETO BREAD RECIPES

COLLAGEN KETO BREAD

This collagen keto bread has zero net carbs per slice. It's dairy-free, grain-free, gluten-free, and best of all, it uses heat-stable, grass-fed collagen protein as its primary ingredient for giving the bread its structure. This keto bread is fluffy, delicious, not overly eggy, and all this with zero net carbs per slice.

Total time: 1hr 30min

Serves: 12

INGREDIENTS:

- ✓ 1/2 cup Unflavored Grass-Fed Collagen Protein
- ✓ 6 tablespoons almond flour (see recipe notes below for nut-free substitute)
- ✓ 5 pastured eggs, separated
- ✓ 1 tablespoon unflavored liquid coconut oil
- ✓ 1 teaspoon aluminum-free baking powder
- ✓ 1 teaspoon xanthan gum (see recipe notes for substitute)
- ✓ Pinch Himalayan pink salt
- ✓ Optional: pinch of stevia

INSTRUCTIONS:

Preheat oven to 325 degrees F.

Generously oil only the bottom part of a standard size (1.5 quart) glass or ceramic loaf dish with coconut oil (or butter or ghee). Or you may use a piece of parchment paper trimmed to fit the bottom of your dish. Not oiling or lining the sides of your dish will allow the bread to attach to the sides and stay lifted while it cools.

In a large bowl, beat the egg whites until stiff peaks form. Set aside.

In a small bowl, whisk the dry ingredients together and set aside. Add the optional pinch of stevia if you're not a fan of eggs. It'll help offset the flavor without adding sweetness to your loaf.

In a small bowl, whisk together the wet ingredients — egg yolks and liquid coconut oil — and set aside.

Add the dry and the wet ingredients to the egg whites and mix until well incorporated. Your batter will be thick and a little gooey.

Pour the batter into the oiled or lined dish and place in the oven.

Bake for 40 minutes. The bread will rise significantly in the oven.

Remove from oven and let it cool completely — about 1 to 2 hours. The bread will sink some and that's OK.

Once the bread is cooled, run the sharp edge of a knife around the edges of the dish to release the loaf.

Slice into 12 even slices.

Important Notes:

Storing Leftovers: Store loosely covered in the refrigerator for up to 5 days.

Reheating: You can eat this bread cold (it stays nice and moist), or bring to room temperature by setting it out on the counter, or pan-sear on the stovetop with ghee or butter. I don't recommend toasting it in a toaster. Although it does work, it's not my preferred method as it has a tendency to dry out too quickly.

Tasting Notes: To set expectations correctly, you should understand that this is not gluten bread nor is it Paleo bread, both of which generally have a fair amount of carbs, often coming from starches and sugars. Rather, this is an extremely low carb/zero carb keto bread alternative. With that said, you may taste eggs, especially if you're not a fan of their flavor.

Additionally, the texture is lighter than gluten bread and won't have the "chew" you may be accustomed to. However, if you're a seasoned keto bread eater, I think you'll find this to be a wonderful option.

Recipe Notes: For those that can't tolerate almond flour, substitute the same amount of coconut flour and add 3 tablespoons of full-fat canned coconut milk (BPA-free) to your ingredients list (you will add coconut milk when instructions call for mixing wet ingredients together). This will increase the net carbs by 1.5 grams per serving, and will make a more dense texture. For keto bread without xanthan gum, substitute with 3/4 tablespoon of konjac flour (also known as glucomannan powder). This will not change the net carb count.

ALMOND FLOUR BREAD

This fluffy and easy almond flour bread has a texture just like wholewheat bread. It's fantastic for sandwiches and toasts well. With low-carb pantry staples like almond flour and Himalayan salt, this keto bread recipe produces a basic loaf with no eggy taste whatsoever. Separating the eggs helps this bread stay fluffy without any yeast — plus, each slice is only 1.25 net carbs. To stay more Bulletproof, simply use grass-fed butter.

Total time: 50min

Serves: 12

INGREDIENTS

- ✓ 2 egg whites at room temperature
- ✓ 2 eggs white & yolk, at room temperature
- ✓ 2 cups / 200g almond flour
- ✓ 1/4 cup / 60g butter melted
- ✓ 4 tbsp / 20g psyllium husks or 2 tbsp. psyllium husk powder
- ✓ 1 1/2 tsp baking powder
- ✓ 1/2 tsp. xanthan gum
- ✓ pinch of salt

✓ 1/2 cup plus 2 tbsp / 140g warm water

INSTRUCTIONS

Preheat your oven to 180 Celsius / 350 Fahrenheit

Beat the 2 eggs and the 2 additional egg whites. (You can reserve the 2 leftover yolks for mayonnaise)

Add the rest of the ingredients and blend until you have a smooth dough. Don't over-mix.

Fill into a lined baking tin (I used a small loaf pan 7 x 3.5 inch / 18 x 9 cm / 450 ml volume) and bake for ca 45 minutes or until a knife inserted comes out clean

Recipe Notes

You can use a regular 9 x 5 inch loaf pan for this almond flour bread recipe. It will come out a bit flatter than your regular toast slice though.

Low carb bread is filling and slices don't need to be the same size as regular wheat bread. That's why I purchased a small loaf pan like this for low carb baking. It's half the size of a regular loaf pan.

Check after 35 minutes - if the top of the bread starts browning too much, cover it with a piece of aluminium paper. This will prevent the top from getting too dark / burning.

LOW CARB KETO BREAD RECIPE

Slice up this Paleo keto bread and pile it high with your favorite sandwich fixings. If you are sensitive to lactose, try this keto bread recipe. Instead of butter, the ingredients list calls for grass-fed ghee, which contains much little to no lactose. With only four other ingredients, you can have this loaf ready to enjoy in well under an hour. Plus, each luscious slice tallies up to 3 net carbs.

This bread also doubles as delicious savory or sweet muffins. Stir in blueberries to make blueberry muffins (keep in mind, however, that the carb count will go up) or chopped jalapeños and nutritional yeast for a spicy muffin with a cheesy twist.

Total time: 55min

Serves: 12

INGREDIENTS

- ✓ 7 large eggs
- ✓ 1/2 cup melted ghee
- ✓ 2 cups almond flour
- ✓ 1 t baking powder
- ✓ 1/4 t sea salt

INSTRUCTIONS

Preheat the oven to 350°F and line a loaf pan with parchment paper overlapping the sides.

In a large mixing bowl, beat the eggs using a hand mixer on high speed for 1 minute. Add the melted ghee and beat until just incorporated.

Reduce the speed to low and gradually add the remaining ingredients until completely mixed and the batter is thick.

Pour the batter into the prepared pan and spread with a spatula. Bake for 40-45 minutes, or until light golden brown on top.

Cool the bread on a cooling rack for 10 minutes before slicing.

PALEO COCONUT BREAD

This paleo keto bread recipe makes a delicious option for coconut lovers. For a low-fuss loaf, blend coconut flour with ingredients like eggs, coconut oil, and salt — then bake away for a sturdy bread with only 1.3 net carbs per serving. Make this recipe totally nut-free (and more Bulletproof) by swapping almond milk with full-fat canned coconut milk.

Total time: 50min

Serves: 10

INGREDIENTS

- ✓ 1/2 cup coconut flour
- ✓ 1/4 tsp salt
- ✓ 1/4 tsp. baking soda
- ✓ 6 eggs
- ✓ ¼ cup coconut oil, melted
- ✓ ¼ unsweetened almond milk

INSTRUCTIONS

Preheat oven to 350°F.

Line an 8×4 inch loaf pan with parchment paper.

In a bowl combine the coconut flour, baking soda and salt.

In another bowl combine the eggs, milk and oil.

Slowly add the wet ingredients into the dry ingredients and mix until combined.

Pour the mixture into the prepared loaf pan.

Bake for 40-50 minutes, or until a toothpick, inserted in the middle comes out clean.

Easy Paleo Keto Bread

Using a blend of almond and coconut flours, this sturdy keto bread will even hold up to freezing. Take 10 minutes to blend flours with baking powder, salt, butter, and egg whites, then bake for an easy loaf that won't turn your kitchen upside down. Stay more Bulletproof and use grass-fed butter in this recipe — each slice will still run you just 1 net carb.

Total time: 1hr 20min

Serves: 18

Basic Ingredients

- ✓ 1 cup Blanched almond flour

- ✓ 1/4 cup Coconut flour

- ✓ 2 tsp. Gluten-free baking powder

- ✓ 1/4 tsp Sea salt

- ✓ 1/3 cup Butter (or 5 tbsp. + 1 tsp; measured solid, then melted; can use coconut oil for dairy-free)

- ✓ 12 large Egg white (~1 1/2 cups, at room temperature)

Optional Ingredients (recommended)

- ✓ 1 1/2 tbsp. Erythritol (can use any sweetener or omit)

- ✓ 1/4 tsp. Xanthan gum (for texture - omit for paleo)

✓ 1/4 tsp. Cream of tartar (to more easily whip egg whites)

INSTRUCTIONS

Preheat the oven to 325 degrees F (163 degrees C). Line an 8 1/2 x 4 1/2 in (22x11 cm) loaf pan with parchment paper, with extra hanging over the sides for easy removal later.

Combine the almond flour, coconut flour, baking powder, erythritol, xanthan gum, and sea salt in a large food processor. Pulse until combined.

Add the melted butter. Pulse, scraping down the sides as needed, until crumbly.

In a very large bowl, use a hand mixer to beat the egg whites and cream of tartar (if using), until stiff peaks form. Make sure the bowl is large enough because the whites will expand a lot.

Add 1/2 of the stiff egg whites to the food processor. Pulse a few times until just combined. Do not over-mix!

Carefully transfer the mixture from the food processor into the bowl with the egg whites, and gently fold until no streaks remain. Do not stir. Fold gently to keep the mixture as fluffy as possible.

Transfer the batter to the lined loaf pan and smooth the top. Push the batter toward the center a bit to round the top.

Bake for about 40 minutes, until the top is golden brown. Tent the top with aluminum foil and bake for another 30-45 minutes, until the top is firm and does not make a squishy sound when pressed. Internal temperature should be 200 degrees. Cool completely before removing from the pan and slicing.

RECIPE NOTES

This recipe was slightly updated in June 2018 to reduce baking temperature to 325 degrees, increase cook time, and better describe signs of doneness. These changes reduce the chance of having an undercooked center.

Check the tips above the recipe card for tips on how to make this the best keto bread recipe for white bread!

EASY CLOUD BREAD

Most iterations of this keto bread recipe include inflammatory cream cheese, but this one uses coconut cream to keep every bite dairy-free. Just like ordinary cloud bread, this recipe makes light and fluffy slices — all with only four ingredients and .4 net carbs per serving.

Total time: 35min

Serves: 10

INGREDIENTS

- ✓ 3 eggs
- ✓ 3 tbsp coconut cream spoon from a refrigerated can of full-fat coconut milk
- ✓ 1/2 tsp baking powder
- ✓ Optional toppings: sea salt black pepper and rosemary or whatever seasonings you like!

INSTRUCTIONS

Firstly, prep everything. Once you start going, you'll need to move quickly so have everything handy. Pre-heat the oven to 325f degrees and arrange a rack in the middle. Line a baking sheet with parchment paper and set aside. Grab your tools: hand mixer (you can use a stand mixer, but I find it to be better for whipping egg whites so I can stay in control), all ingredients, any additional seasonings, two mixing bowls (the larger one should be used for egg whites), a large spoon to scoop and drop the bread with.

Using a full-fat can of coconut milk that has been refrigerated overnight or several hours, spoon out the top coconut cream and add to the smaller bowl.

Separate eggs into the two bowls, adding the yolk to the bowl with the cream and be careful to not let the yolk get into the whites in the larger bowl.

Using a hand mixer, beat the yolk and cream together first until nice and creamy, make sure there are no clumps of coconut left.

Wash your whisks well and dry them.

Add the baking powder into the whites and start beating on medium with the hand mixer for a few minutes, moving around and you'll see it get firmer. Keep going for a few minutes, you want to get it as thick as you can with stiff peaks. The thicker the better. Just don't over-do it. Once you can stop and dip the whisks in leaving peaks behind, you're ready.

Quickly and carefully add the yolk-coconut mixture into the whites, folding with a spatula, careful not to deflate too much. Keep going until everything is well combined but still fluffy.

Now you can grab your spoon and start dropping your batter down on the baking sheet. Keep going as quickly and carefully as you can, or it will start to melt. They should look pillow-y.

Steadily add your baking sheet to the middle rack in the oven and bake for approx. 20-25 minutes. You should be able to scoop them up with your spatula and see a fluffy top and a flat bottom. Store in the fridge for about a week or freeze.

MACADAMIA NUT BREAD

This keto bread recipe creates a perfect outer crust and soft crumb, thanks to high-fat macadamia nuts ground right into the batter. Blend nuts with eggs, coconut flour, baking soda, and apple cider vinegar, then bake. That's it! Per slice, each serving runs 1 net carb — just make sure you avoid eating macadamias too often to stay Bulletproof.

Total time: 50min

Serves: 10

INGREDIENTS

- ✓ 5 oz macadamia nuts I used the Royal Hawaiian brand
- ✓ 5 large eggs
- ✓ 1/4 cup coconut flour (28 g)
- ✓ 1/2 teaspoon baking soda
- ✓ 1/2 teaspoon apple cider vinegar

INSTRUCTIONS

Preheat oven to 350F.

To a blender or food processor, add macadamia nuts and pulse until it becomes a nut butter. If your blender does not do a good job without liquid, add in eggs one at a time until the consistency is that of a nut butter.

Scrape down sides of blender or food processor, and add in the remaining eggs. Blend until well-incorporated.

Add in coconut flour, baking soda and apple cider vinegar and pulse until incorporated.

Grease a standard-size bread pan and add in batter. Smooth surface of batter and place on bottom rack of oven for 30-40 minutes, or until the top is golden brown.

Remove from oven and allow to cool in pan for 15-20 minutes before removing.

Will store in an air-tight container at room temperature for 3-4 days at room temperature, or for one week in the fridge.

Low-Carb Garlic & Herb Focaccia

A combination of baking soda, lemon juice, and baking powder eliminates the need for yeast in this bubbly keto bread recipe. With tons of Italian seasonings, olive oil, and flaky salt sprinkled on top, you'll want to include this loaf with every meal. Each generous slice is 3 net carbs — and to stay more Bulletproof, simply avoid eating garlic and xanthan gum too often.

Total time: 30min

Serves: 8

INGREDIENTS

Dry Ingredients

- ✓ 1 cup Almond Flour
- ✓ ¼ cup Coconut Flour
- ✓ ½ tsp. Xanthan Gum
- ✓ 1 tsp. Garlic Powder
- ✓ 1 tsp. Flaky Salt
- ✓ ½ tsp. Baking Soda
- ✓ ½ tsp. Baking Powder

Wet Ingredients

- ✓ 2 eggs

- ✓ 1 tbsp. Lemon Juice

- ✓ 2 tsp Olive oil + 2 tbsp. Olive Oil to drizzle

- ✓ Top with Italian Seasoning and TONS of flaky salt!

INSTRUCTIONS

Heat oven to 350 and line a baking tray or 8-inch round pan with parchment.

Whisk together the dry ingredients making sure there are no lumps.

Beat the egg, lemon juice, and oil until combined.

Mix the wet and the dry together, working quickly, and scoop the dough into your pan.

Make sure not to mix the wet and dry until you are ready to put the bread in the oven because the leavening reaction begins once it is mixed!!!

Smooth the top and edges with a spatula dipped in water (or your hands) then use your finger to dimple the dough. Don't be afraid to go deep on the dimples! Again, a little water keeps it from sticking.

Bake covered for about 10 minutes. Drizzle with Olive Oil bake for an additional 10-15 minutes uncovering to brown gently.

Top with more flaky salt, olive oil (optional), a dash of Italian seasoning and fresh basil. Let cool completely before slicing for optimal texture!!

Notes

3g Net Carbs per big long slice.

You can also cut it into squares and you'd just want to adjust how many servings you get vs. the macros

CAULIFLOWER BREAD WITH GARLIC & HERBS

Sneak some veggies into your keto bread with this simple, flavorful recipe. A combination of riced cauliflower and coconut flour makes a convincing substitute for starchy bread ingredients, while sea salt and herbs add a savory touch. To stay Bulletproof on this 3-carb bread, use grass-fed butter and avoid eating garlic too often.

Total time: 1hr 10min

Serves: 12

INGREDIENTS

- ✓ 3 c. riced cauliflower
- ✓ 6 eggs, separated
- ✓ 1 1/4 c. almond flour
- ✓ 1 tbsp. baking powder
- ✓ 1 tsp.. kosher salt
- ✓ 6 tbsp.. melted butter
- ✓ 5 cloves garlic, minced
- ✓ 1 tbsp.. chopped thyme
- ✓ 1 tbsp.. parsley, chopped
- ✓ Parmesan, for serving

INSTRUCTIONS

Preheat oven to 350° and line a 9-x-5" loaf pan with parchment paper. In a medium bowl, microwave cauliflower for 3 to 4 minutes or until soft and tender. Let cool. When cool enough to handle, transfer cauliflower to a clean kitchen towel and squeeze to release as much moisture as possible.

In a medium bowl, beat egg whites until stiff peaks form. Set aside.

In a large bowl, whisk together almond flour, baking powder, salt, egg yolks, melted butter, garlic and about a quarter of the whipped egg whites. Beat until well combined, then stir in microwaved cauliflower. Fold in the remaining egg whites and mix until just incorporated. (Mixture should be fluffy.) Fold in the thyme and most of the parsley (save some for topping).

Transfer batter to the lined loaf pan and sprinkle with more herbs. Bake until the top is golden, about 45 to 50 minutes. Let cool completely before slicing.

Sprinkle slices with Parmesan and more parsley.

KETO BREAD RECIPES: FLATBREADS AND TORTILLAS

15-MINUTE GRAIN-FREE TORTILLAS

Even without the gluten of a traditional tortilla, this keto bread recipe creates a soft and pliable alternative perfect for all your favorite taco fillings. Almond and coconut flours keep carbs to a minimum, while xanthan gum holds everything together. Each tortilla tallies up to 2 net carbs, and takes only five minutes to cook. No Bulletproof substitutions needed — just avoid eating xanthan gum too often.

Total time: 15min

Serves: 8

INGREDIENTS

- ✓ 96 g almond flour
- ✓ 24 g coconut flour
- ✓ 2 teaspoons xanthan gum
- ✓ 1 teaspoon baking powder
- ✓ 1/4 teaspoon kosher salt
- ✓ 2 teaspoons apple cider vinegar
- ✓ 1 egg lightly beaten

✓ 3 teaspoons water

INSTRUCTIONS

Add almond flour, coconut flour, xanthan gum, baking powder and salt to food processor. Pulse until thoroughly combined. Note: You can alternatively whisk everything in a large bowl and use a hand or stand mixer for the following steps.

Pour in apple cider vinegar with the food processor running. Once it has distributed evenly, pour in the egg. Followed by the water. Stop the food processor once the dough forms into a ball. The dough will be sticky to touch.

Wrap dough in cling film and knead it through the plastic for a minute or two. Think of it a bit like a stress ball. Allow dough to rest for 10 minutes (and up to three days in the fridge).

Heat up a skillet (preferably) or pan over medium heat. You can test the heat by sprinkling a few water droplets, if the drops evaporate immediately your pan is too hot. The droplets should 'run' through the skillet.

Break the dough into eight 1" balls (26g each). Roll out between two sheets of parchment or waxed paper with a rolling pin or using a tortilla press (easier!) until each round is 5-inches in diameter.

Transfer to skillet and cook over medium heat for just 3-6 seconds (very important). Flip it over immediately (using a thin spatula or knife), and continue to cook until just lightly golden on each side (though with the traditional charred marks), 30 to 40 seconds. The key is not to overcook them, as they will no longer be pliable or puff up.

Keep them warm wrapped in kitchen cloth until serving. To rewarm, heat briefly on both sides, until just warm (less than a minute).

These tortillas are best eaten straight away. But feel free to keep some dough handy in your fridge for up to three days, and they also freeze well for up to three months.

RECIPE NOTES

One (very important!!) thing: when cooking, coconut flour burns rather rapidly. So while this does help you to get the traditional charred marks of flour tortillas, you do need to keep an eye out for them to keep them from burning. Having said that, you do want your skillet to be very hot in order for the tortillas to cook quickly (in under a minute) and stay pliable. Like any tortilla, if the heat is not high enough it will harden and crack.

COCONUT FLOUR FLATBREAD

Use this keto bread for wraps, dips, curries, and anywhere else you'd normally use a naan-style bread. This recipe creates tasty, pliable bread with no eggs and only 2.6 net carbs per serving. To keep it more Bulletproof, swap olive oil with avocado oil or coconut oil, and avoid eating psyllium husk too often.

Total time: 15min

Serves: 6

INGREDIENTS

- ✓ 2 tablespoons psyllium husk (9g)

- ✓ 1/2 cup coconut flour fine, fresh, no lumps (60g)

- ✓ 1 cup lukewarm water (240ml)

- ✓ 1 tablespoon olive oil (15ml)

- ✓ 1/4 teaspoons baking soda

- ✓ 1/4 teaspoons salt - optional

COOKING

- ✓ 1 teaspoon olive oil to rub/oil the nonstick pan

INSTRUCTIONS

MAKE THE DOUGH

In a medium mixing bowl, combine the psyllium husk and coconut flour (if lumps are in your flour use a fork to smash them BEFORE measuring the flour, amount must be precise).

Add in the lukewarm water (I used tap water about 40C/bath temperature), olive oil, and baking soda. Give a good stir with a spatula, then use your hands to knead the dough. Add salt now if you want. I never add the salt in contact with baking soda to avoid deactivating the leaving agent.

Knead for 1 minute. The dough is moist and it gets softer and slightly dryer as you go. It should come together easily to form a dough as on my picture. If not, too sticky, add more husk, 1/2 teaspoon at a time, knead for 30 sec and see how it goes. The dough will always be a bit moist, but it shouldn't stick to your hands at all. It must come together as a dough.

Set aside 10 minute in the mixing bowl.

Now the dough must be soft, elastic and hold well together, it is ready to roll.

ROLL/ SHAPE THE FLATBREAD

Cut the dough into 4 even pieces, roll each piece into a small ball.

Place one of the dough balls between two pieces of parchment paper, press the ball with your hand palm to stick it well to the paper and start rolling it with a rolling pin as thin as you like a bread. My breads are 20 cm diameter (8 inches) and I made 6 flatbread with this recipe.

Un peel the first layer of parchment paper from your flatbread. Use a lid to cut out round flatbread. Keep the outside dough to reform a ball and roll more flatbread - that is how I make 2 extra flatbread from the 4 balls above!

COOK IN NON STICK PAN

Warm a non stick tefal crepe/ pancake pan under medium/high heat- or use any nonstick pan of your choice, the one you would use for your pancakes.

Add one teaspoon of olive oil or vegetable oil of your choice onto a piece of absorbent paper. Rub the surface of the pan to make sure it is slightly oiled. Don't leave any drops of oil or the bread will fry!

Flip over the flatbread on the hot pan and peel off the last piece of parchment paper carefully.

Cook for 2-3 minutes on the first side, flip over using a spatula and cook for 1-2 more minute on the other side.

Cool down the flatbread on a plate and use as a sandwich wrap later or enjoy hot as a side dish. I recommend a drizzle of olive oil, crushed garlic and herbs before serving ! (optional but delish!)

Repeat the rolling, cooking for the next 3 flatbread. Make sure you rub the oiled absorbent paper onto the saucepan each time to avoid the bread to stick to the pan.

Store in the pantry in an airtight box or on a plate covered with plastic wrap to keep them soft, for up to 3 days.

Rewarm in the same pan or if you want to give them a little crisp rewarm in the hot oven on a baking sheet for 1-2 minutes at 150C.

Blue color? Some psyllium husk bran turns out blue or purple when cooked. Mine doesn't (see here) try different brand to find out the one that is right for you. If your wraps turns out blue or purple, you can still eat the wraps, the color is a natural reaction from the husk, that is all. It doesn't change the flavor or properties of the recipe.

Recipe size: I made 6 flatbread with this recipe - I reused the border of the 4 fltbread cut into round shape to reform 2 extra flatbread. Feel free to double up the recipe to make more flatbread!

Storage: store in the pantry up to 3 days onto a plate covered with plastic wrap to keep them soft or in the fridge up to 5 days.

Rewarm tips: They are softer when cold and stored for a few days. I rewarm mine in the pan or in a hot oven or if I make a sandwich wrap, in a toaster press.

Freeze: You can freeze them as you would freeze regular flatbread. Rewarm in the oven or in a sandwich toaster to give them a little crisp.

Net carbs is carbs minus fibre, 2.6 g net carbs per flatbread in this recipe.

CAULIFLOWER TORTILLAS

This paleo, keto bread alternative uses cauliflower as a base for flexible, flavorful tortillas. Squeezing the moisture out of the riced cauliflower, plus adding eggs, keeps these tortillas sturdy enough for taco fillings or wraps. To stay more Bulletproof, steam cauliflower instead of microwaving.

Total time: 50min

Serves: 6

INGREDIENTS

- ✓ 3/4 large head cauliflower (or two cups riced)
- ✓ 2 large eggs (Vegans, sub flax eggs)
- ✓ 1/4 cup chopped fresh cilantro
- ✓ 1/2 medium lime, juiced and zested
- ✓ Salt & pepper, to taste

INSTRUCTIONS

Preheat the oven to 375 degrees F., and line a baking sheet with parchment paper.

Trim the cauliflower, cut it into small, uniform pieces, and pulse in a food processor in batches until you get a couscous-like consistency. The finely riced cauliflower should make about 2 cups packed.

Place the cauliflower in a microwave-safe bowl and microwave for 2 minutes, then stir and microwave again for another 2 minutes. If you don't use a microwave, a steamer works just as well. Place the cauliflower in a fine cheesecloth or thin dishtowel and squeeze out as much liquid as possible, being careful not to burn yourself. Dishwashing gloves are suggested as it is very hot.

In a medium bowl, whisk the eggs. Add in cauliflower, cilantro, lime, salt and pepper. Mix until well combined. Use your hands to shape 6 small "tortillas" on the parchment paper.

Bake for 10 minutes, carefully flip each tortilla, and return to the oven for an additional 5 to 7 minutes, or until completely set. Place tortillas on a wire rack to cool slightly.

Heat a medium-sized skillet on medium. Place a baked tortilla in the pan, pressing down slightly, and brown for 1 to 2 minutes on each side. Repeat with remaining tortillas.

RECIPE NOTES

*WEIGHT WATCHERS POINTS PER TORTILLA: Freestyle SmartPoints: 0, SmartPoints: 1, Points Plus: 1, Old Points Program: 1

*You can munch these by themselves, make quesadillas with them, or add some taco filling and fold it like a taco.

*Some people have mentioned in the comments that they've had success using already riced cauliflower instead of processing a head of cauliflower.

*Leftover tortillas should freeze well for you.

BUTTERY & SOFT SKILLET FLATBREAD

No oven, no problem: You can still make keto bread right from your skillet with this recipe. Since it uses simple ingredients and cooks in batches from your stovetop, you won't have to wait long for bread to cool before devouring it. To stay Bulletproof, use grass-fed butter and avoid eating too much xanthan gum.

Total time: 7 min

Serves: 4

INGREDIENTS

- ✓ 1 cup Almond Flour
- ✓ 2 tbsp Coconut Flour
- ✓ 2 tsp Xanthan Gum
- ✓ ½ tsp. Baking Powder
- ✓ ½ tsp. Falk Salt + more to garnish
- ✓ 1 Whole Egg + 1 Egg White
- ✓ 1 tbsp. Water
- ✓ 1 tbsp. Oil for frying
- ✓ 1 tbsp. melted Butter-for slathering

INSTRUCTIONS

Whisk together the dry ingredients (flours, xanthan gum, baking powder, salt) until well combined.

Add the egg and egg white and beat gently into the flour to incorporate. The dough will begin to form.

Add the tablespoon of water and begin to work the dough to allow the flour and xanthan gum to absorb the moisture.

Cut the dough in 4 equal parts and press each section out with cling wrap. Watch the video for instructions!

Heat a large skillet over medium heat and add oil.

Fry each flatbread for about 1 min on each side.

Brush with butter (while hot) and garnish with salt and chopped parsley.

Notes:

NET Carbs = 4g

*If you want a smaller portion, just cut the dough into 5 balls instead of 4!

KETO BREAD ROLLS, BAGELS & BUNS

FLUFFY KETO BUNS

When you crave a pillowy-soft roll for burgers, sandwiches, and bread baskets, make this keto bread recipe. Eggs, coconut flour, and psyllium husk make up the bulk of the dough before baking into perfectly spongy buns — all at 6 net carbs apiece.

Total time: 50min

Serves: 4

INGREDIENTS:

- ✓ 1/4 cup coconut flour

- ✓ 2 tablespoons ground psyllium husks

- ✓ 4 egg whites

- ✓ 2 egg yolks

- ✓ 1 teaspoon paleo baking powder

- ✓ 1/2 tablespoon apple cider vinegar

- ✓ 1 cup water

- ✓ 1 teaspoon dried oregano (optional)

- ✓ 1 teaspoon dried thyme (optional)

- ✓ Salt and pepper to taste

INSTRUCTIONS:

Preheat your oven to 350 degrees. Line a baking sheet with parchment paper.

With a hand mixer or whisk, beat the egg whites until they form a foam with stiff peaks. Set aside.

Mix all remaining ingredients in a separate bowl. Gently fold in the egg whites.

Form four thick, evenly sized rolls from your dough and place on the baking sheet. (Thickness is important so buns don't flatten.)

Bake for 40 minutes, or until cooked all the way through. If you cut one open and it still is moist, place them (even the one you have cut open) back in the oven for a few more minutes.

Remove from your oven and serve warm.

30-MINUTE DROP BISCUITS

This "lazy" keto bread recipe is anything but boring: Crumbling the butter directly into the dough creates moist and tender biscuits for all your sweet and savory recipes. Plus, this recipe takes 30 minutes from start to finish and keeps each biscuit macro-friendly at 3 net carbs. Stay more Bulletproof and use the sour cream and whey protein swaps suggested in the recipe, plus avoid eating flaxseed too often.

Total time: 30min

Serves: 6

INGREDIENTS

- ✓ 1 egg

- ✓ 77 g sour cream or coconut cream + 2 tsp. apple cider vinegar, at room temp

- ✓ 2 tablespoons water

- ✓ 1 tablespoon apple cider vinegar

- ✓ 96 g almond flour

- ✓ 63 g golden flaxseed meal or psyllium husk, finely ground

- ✓ 21 g coconut flour

- ✓ 20 g whey protein isolate or more almond flour

- ✓ 3 1/2 teaspoons baking powder

- ✓ 1 teaspoon xanthan gum or 1 TBS. flaxseed meal

- ✓ 1/2 teaspoon kosher salt

- ✓ 112 g organic grass-fed butter or 7 TBS. ghee/coconut oil

INSTRUCTIONS

Preheat oven to 450°F/230°C. Line a baking tray with parchment paper or a baking mat.

Add eggs, sour (or coconut) cream, water and apple cider vinegar to a medium bowl and whisk for a minute or two until fully mixed. Set aside.

Add almond flour, flaxseed meal, coconut flour, whey protein, baking powder, xanthan gum (or more flax) and kosher salt to a food processor and pulse until very thoroughly combined.

Add in the butter and pulse a few times until pea-sized. Pour in the egg and cream mixture, pulsing until combined. The dough will be very shaggy.

Drop 6 rounds of dough onto the prepared baking tray. Brush with melted butter and bake for 15-20 minutes until deep golden. Allow to cool for 10 minutes before serving. These guys keep well, stored in an airtight container at room temperature, for 3-4 days.

You can freeze the shaped biscuit dough for 1-2 months, and bake straight from the freezer as needed.

RECIPE NOTES

Please see post for deets, possible subs, and methodology without a food processor.

We found each batch to yield 6 biscuits, and nutrition facts were estimated per biscuit.

ROSEMARY KETO BAGELS

Use this keto bread recipe to create chewy and dense bagels with less than 5 net carbs. Almond flour blends with binders like eggs, xanthan gum, and psyllium husk for a sturdy base, while chopped rosemary adds an herby finish. Avoid eating xanthan gum and psyllium too often to stay more Bulletproof.

Total time: 55min

Serves: 4

INGREDIENTS:

- ✓ 1 1/2 cups almond flour
- ✓ 3/4 teaspoon baking soda
- ✓ 3/4 teaspoon xanthan gum
- ✓ 1/4 teaspoon salt
- ✓ 3 tablespoons psyllium husk powder
- ✓ 1 whole egg
- ✓ 3 egg whites
- ✓ 1/2 cup warm water
- ✓ 1 tablespoon rosemary, chopped
- ✓ Avocado oil

INSTRUCTIONS:

Preheat oven to 250F.

Mix almond flour, xanthan gum, baking soda and salt together in a bowl.

In a separate bowl, whisk eggs and warm water together. Stir in psyllium husk until there are no clumps.

Add liquid ingredients to dry ingredients.

Coat bagel mold with avocado oil.

Press dough into mold.

Sprinkle rosemary on top.

Place in oven and bake for 45 minutes.

Remove and cool for 15 minutes before slicing.

TURMERIC CAULIFLOWER BUNS

Cauliflower makes a delicious replacement in low-carb recipes, and this keto bread is no exception. Riced cauliflower blends with coconut flour and anti-inflammatory turmeric to create hot and fluffy buns with no veggie taste. To stay more Bulletproof, steam cauliflower instead of microwaving and skip the black pepper.

Total time: 60min

Serves: 6

INGREDIENTS

- ✓ 1 medium head of cauliflower or about 2 cups of firmly packed cauliflower rice (see directions for making the cauliflower rice)

- ✓ 2 eggs

- ✓ 2 tablespoons coconut flour

- ✓ ¼ teaspoon ground turmeric

- ✓ Pinch each of salt and pepper

INSTRUCTIONS

Preheat oven to 400°F.

Line a baking sheet with parchment paper and set aside.

Take your cauliflower and use a sharp knife to cut off the base. Pull off any green parts and use your hands to break the cauliflower into florets. Give the florets a quick rinse and pat dry.

Next, make cauliflower rice by placing the florets into the bowl of a food processor with the "S" blade. Pulse for about 30 seconds until the cauliflower is about the size of rice. You should have about two cups of firmly packed cauliflower rice.

Place the cauliflower rice into a microwavable-safe bowl with about a teaspoon of water. Cover with plastic wrap and poke a few holes to let the steam escape. Microwave the cauliflower rice for about 3 minutes. Alternatively, you can steam the cauliflower rice on the stovetop in a steamer basket.

Uncover the bowl and let the cauliflower rice cool for about 5 minutes. Then, use a large spoon to put the cauliflower rice into a nut milk bag or a clean dish towel. Squeeze the excess moisture out, being careful not to burn your hands.

Pour the cauliflower rice into a medium mixing bowl and stir in the eggs, turmeric, and a pinch of salt and black pepper.

Use your hands to form the mixture into 6 buns, placing them on the baking sheet.

Bake for 25-30 minutes or until the top becomes slightly browned.

The cauliflower buns are best served hot right out of the oven. They do not refrigerate or re-heat well (they will get mushy), but they are so delicious that you'll no doubt eat them right away!

Low-Carb Almond Flour Biscuits

With five ingredients and 10 minutes of prep, this keto bread proves anyone can make keto bread. This recipe makes buttery rolls with almond flour as the main ingredient, and each one runs only 2 net carbs. Keep this recipe more Bulletproof with grass-fed butter or ghee.

Total time: 25min

Serves: 12

INGREDIENTS

- ✓ 2 cup Blanched almond flour
- ✓ 2 tsp. Gluten-free baking powder
- ✓ 1/2 tsp. Sea salt
- ✓ 2 large Egg (beaten)
- ✓ 1/3 cup Butter (measured solid, then melted; can use ghee or coconut oil for dairy-free)

INSTRUCTIONS

Preheat the oven to 350 degrees F (177 degrees C). Line a baking sheet with parchment paper.

Mix dry ingredients together in a large bowl. Stir in wet ingredients.

Scoop tablespoonfuls of the dough onto the lined baking sheet (a cookie scoop is the fastest way). Form into rounded biscuit shapes (flatten slightly with your fingers).

Bake for about 15 minutes, until firm and golden. Cool on the baking sheet.

Cranberry Jalapeño "Cornbread" Muffins

This keto bread recipe delivers sweet heat with no corn whatsoever — instead, it uses a blend of coconut flour and sweetener to capture the same taste and texture for about 3 net carbs per serving. Add fresh cranberries and jalapeño slices for a fun twist that pairs well with holiday meals. To keep this recipe more Bulletproof, use grass-fed butter, swap almond milk with full-fat canned coconut milk, and skip the peppers if you have a nightshade sensitivity.

Total time: 40min

Serves: 12

INGREDIENTS

- ✓ 1 cup coconut flour (I used Bob's Red Mill)
- ✓ 1/3 cup Swerve Sweetener or other erythritol
- ✓ 1 tbsp baking powder
- ✓ 1/2 tsp. salt
- ✓ 7 large eggs, lightly beaten
- ✓ 1 cup unsweetened almond milk
- ✓ 1/2 cup butter, melted OR avocado oil
- ✓ 1/2 tsp. vanilla
- ✓ 1 cup fresh cranberries, cut in half

- ✓ 3 tbsp. minced jalapeño peppers
- ✓ 1 jalapeño, seeds removed, sliced into 12 slices, for garnish

INSTRUCTIONS

Preheat oven to 325F and grease a muffin tin well or line with paper liners.

In a medium bowl, whisk together coconut flour, sweetener, baking powder and salt. Break up any clumps with the back of a fork.

Stir in eggs, melted butter and almond milk and stir vigorously. Stir in vanilla extract and continue to stir until mixture is smooth and well combined. Stir in chopped cranberries and jalapeños.

Divide batter evenly among prepared muffin cups and place one slice of jalapeño on top of each.

Bake 25 to 30 minutes or until tops are set and a tester inserted in the center comes out clean. Let cool 10 minutes in pan, then transfer to a wire rack to cool completely.

KETO BAGELS

Unlike other low-carb bagels that require conventional cheese to bind them together, this keto bread recipe uses psyllium husk to create the same dense texture. You may want to enjoy these bagels split in half, since each one contains 7 net carbs. Keep every bite more Bulletproof and use grass-fed ghee, swap white vinegar for apple cider vinegar, trade olive oil for avocado oil, and avoid eating psyllium, garlic, or sesame seeds too often.

Total time: 30min

Serves: 2 bagels

INGREDIENTS

- ✓ 1 cup (120 g) of almond flour
- ✓ 1/4 cup (28 g) of coconut flour
- ✓ 1 Tablespoon (7 g) of psyllium husk powder
- ✓ 1 teaspoon (2 g) of baking powder
- ✓ 1 teaspoon (3 g) of garlic powder
- ✓ Pinch salt
- ✓ 2 medium eggs (88 g)
- ✓ 2 teaspoons (10 ml) of white wine vinegar
- ✓ 2 1/2 Tablespoons (38 ml) of ghee, melted

✓ 1 Tablespoon (15 ml) of olive oil

✓ 1 teaspoon (5 g) of sesame seeds

INSTRUCTIONS

Preheat the oven to 320°F (160°C).

Combine the almond flour, coconut flour, psyllium husk powder, baking powder, garlic powder and salt in a bowl.

In a separate bowl, whisk the eggs and vinegar together. Slowly drizzle in the melted ghee (which should not be piping hot) and whisk in well.

Add the wet mixture to the dry mixture and use a wooden spoon to combine well. Leave to sit for 2-3 minutes.

Divide the mixture into 4 equal-sized portions. Using your hands, shape the mixture into a round shape and place onto a tray lined with parchment paper. Use a small spoon or apple corer to make the center hole.

Brush the tops with olive oil and scatter over the sesame seeds. Bake in the oven for 20-25 minutes until cooked through. Allow to cool slightly before enjoying!

KETO BREAD RECIPES: PIZZA CRUST

KETO BREAKFAST PIZZA

While this recipe includes breakfast toppings like smoked salmon and eggs, you can use the keto bread base for savory pizzas as well. Using a blend of riced cauliflower, coconut flour, and psyllium husk, this recipe holds up well to even the heaviest pizza toppings. Plus, each filling serving runs you 7 net carbs.

Total time: 25min

Serves: 2

INGREDIENTS:

- ✓ 2 cups grated cauliflower
- ✓ 2 tablespoons coconut flour
- ✓ 1/2 teaspoon salt
- ✓ 4 eggs
- ✓ 1 tablespoon psyllium husk powder (Use a mold-free brand like this one)
- ✓ Toppings: smoked Salmon, avocado, herbs, spinach, olive oil

INSTRUCTIONS:

Preheat the oven to 350 degrees. Line a pizza tray or sheet pan with parchment.

In a mixing bowl, add all ingredients except toppings and mix until combined. Set aside for 5 minutes to allow coconut flour and psyllium husk to absorb liquid and thicken up.

Carefully pour the breakfast pizza base onto the pan. Use your hands to mold it into a round, even pizza crust.

Bake for 15 minutes, or until golden brown and fully cooked.

Remove from the oven and top breakfast pizza with your chosen toppings. Serve warm.

Note on ingredients: Heavy fibers like psyllium husk can sit undigested in our guts, feeding bad microbes. In large amounts, it can also cause GI distress. Use high-quality psyllium husk whenever possible, consume only occasionally, and get more of your fiber from whole vegetables.

COCONUT FLOUR PIZZA CRUST

Make this keto bread pizza base crispy and thin, or roll it into a thicker, fluffier crust — no matter how you prepare it, this recipe cuts out all dairy, grains, and gluten for a total of 6 net carbs. Coconut flour and psyllium creates a firm texture, while apple cider vinegar lends a tangy flavor. To stay more Bulletproof, avoid eating garlic and psyllium husk too often.

Total time: 35min

Serves: 6

INGREDIENTS

- ✓ 3/4 cup coconut flour clumps removed
- ✓ 3 tablespoons psyllium husk powder
- ✓ 1 teaspoon garlic powder
- ✓ 1/2 teaspoon Salt I love this Himalayan pink salt
- ✓ 1 teaspoon apple cider vinegar
- ✓ 1/2 teaspoon baking soda
- ✓ 3 eggs
- ✓ 1 cup boiling water

INSTRUCTIONS

Preheat oven to 350F.

Mix coconut flour with psyllium husk powder, garlic powder and salt until fully-incorporated.

Add in apple cider vinegar, baking soda and eggs. Mix together.

Mix boiling water in, and stir until incorporated. If the dough is too sticky, add in more coconut flour until it is the desired consistency. The dough will naturally be kind of sticky though, so you may want to use wet fingers to spread out the dough.

Spread dough out on a baking sheet to the desired thickness. I like mine to be pretty thin, so my dough usually covers the entire baking sheet.

Place in a preheated oven for 15-20 minutes, or until edges begin to brown.

Top with sauce, cheese and desired toppings and place back in the oven until the cheese is melted.

15-MINUTE STOVE TOP PIZZA CRUST

In less time than it takes to order delivery, you can have this keto bread base ready to enjoy — plus, it requires no baking! A quick dough made from almond and coconut flours, xanthan gum, and egg, then sizzles in your skillet before taking on your favorite toppings. To keep this 2-carb pizza crust more Bulletproof, avoid eating xanthan gum too often.

Total time: 15min

Serves: 6

INGREDIENTS

FOR THE KETO PIZZA DOUGH:

- ✓ 96 g almond flour
- ✓ 24 g coconut flour
- ✓ 2 teaspoons xanthan gum
- ✓ 2 teaspoons baking powder
- ✓ 1/4 teaspoon kosher salt depending on whether sweet or savory
- ✓ 2 teaspoons apple cider vinegar
- ✓ 1 egg lightly beaten
- ✓ 5 teaspoons water as needed

TOPPING SUGGESTIONS:

- ✓ keto marinara sauce

- ✓ mozzarella cheese

- ✓ pepperoni or salami

- ✓ fresh basil

INSTRUCTIONS

FOR THE KETO DOUGH:

Add almond flour, coconut flour, xanthan gum, baking powder and salt to food processor. Pulse until thoroughly combined.

Pour in apple cider vinegar with the food processor running. Once it has distributed evenly, pour in the egg. Followed by the water, adding just enough for it to come together into a ball. The dough will be sticky to the touch from the xanthan gum, but still sturdy.

Wrap dough in plastic wrap and knead it through the plastic for a minute or two. Think of it a bit like a stress ball. The dough should be smooth and not significantly cracked (a couple here and there are fine). In which case get it back to the food processor and add in more water 1 teaspoon at a time. Allow dough to rest for 10 minutes at room temperature (and up to 5 days in the fridge).

If cooking on the stove top: heat up a skillet or pan over medium/high heat while your dough rests (you want the pan to be very hot!). If using the oven: heat up a pizza stone, skillet or baking tray in the oven at 350°F/180°C. The premise is you need to blind cook/bake the crust first on both sides without toppings on a very hot surface.

Roll out dough between two sheets of parchment paper with a rolling pin. You can play with thickness here, but we like to roll it out nice and thin (roughly 12 inches in diameter) and fold over the edges (pressing down with wet fingertips).

Cook the pizza crust in your pre-heated skillet or pan, top-side down first, until blistered (about 2 minutes, depending on your skillet and heat). Lower heat to medium/low, flip over your pizza crust, add toppings of choice and cover with a lid. Alternatively you can always transfer it to your oven on grill to finish off the pizza.

Serve right away. Alternatively, note that the dough can be kept in the fridge for about 5 days. So you can make individual mini pizzettes throughout the week.

3-Ingredient Mini Paleo Pizza Crusts

This stovetop keto bread base takes an even more minimal approach. Combine almond or coconut flours with egg whites and baking powder, then cook on your stove top for a chewy and sturdy crust. Skip the optional black pepper to stay more Bulletproof.

Serves: 4

INGREDIENTS

For the coconut flour option

- ✓ 8 large egg whites for thicker bases, use 5 whole eggs and 3 egg whites
- ✓ 1/4 cup coconut flour sifted
- ✓ 1/2 tsp. baking powder
- ✓ Spices of choice salt, pepper, Italian spices
- ✓ Extra coconut flour to dust very lightly

For the almond flour option

- ✓ 8 large egg whites
- ✓ 1/2 cup almond flour
- ✓ 1/2 tsp. baking powder
- ✓ Spices of choice salt, pepper, Italian spices

- ✓ For the pizza sauce
- ✓ 1/2 cup Mutti tomato sauce
- ✓ 2 cloves garlic crushed
- ✓ 1/4 tsp. sea salt
- ✓ 1 tsp. dried basil

INSTRUCTIONS

To make the pizza bases/crusts

In a large mixing bowl, whisk the eggs/egg whites until opaque. Sift in the coconut flour or almond flour and whisk very well until clumps are removed. Add the baking powder, mixed spices and continue to whisk until completely combined.

On low heat, heat up a small pan and grease lightly.

Once frying pan is hot, pour the batter in the pan and ensure it is fully coated. Cover the pan with a lid/tray for 3-4 minutes or until bubbles start to appear on top. Flip, cook for an extra 2 minutes and remove from pan- Keep an eye on this, as it can burn out pretty quickly.

Continue until all the batter is used up.

Allow pizza bases to cool. Once cool, use a skewer and poke holes roughly over the top, for even cooking. Dust very lightly with a dash of coconut flour.

To make the sauce

Combine all the ingredients together and let sit at room temperature for at least 30 minutes- This thickens up.

Notes:

For a crispy pizza base, bake in the oven for 3-4 minutes prior to adding your toppings. If you want to freeze them, allow pizza bases to cool completely before topping with a dash of coconut flour and a thin layer of pizza sauce. Ensure each pizza base is divided with parchment paper before placing in the freezer.

KETO BREAD RECIPES: DESSERT BREADS

KETO ZUCCHINI BREAD WITH WALNUTS

This moist and nutty keto bread recipe incorporates wholesome keto ingredients like shredded zucchini, almond flour, and spices. Bake your batter for a sweet loaf under 3 net carbs. Swap olive oil with grass-fed ghee, use Ceylon cinnamon, and skip the nutmeg to stay more Bulletproof.

Total time: 60min

Serves: 15

INGREDIENTS

- ✓ 3 large eggs
- ✓ ½ cup olive oil
- ✓ 1 teaspoon vanilla extract
- ✓ 2 1/2 cups almond flour
- ✓ 1 1/2 cups erythritol
- ✓ ½ teaspoon salt
- ✓ 1 1/2 teaspoons baking powder
- ✓ ½ teaspoon nutmeg
- ✓ 1 teaspoon ground cinnamon

- ✓ ¼ teaspoon ground ginger

- ✓ 1 cup grated zucchini

- ✓ ½ cup chopped walnuts

INSTRUCTIONS

Preheat oven to 350°F. Whisk together the eggs, oil, and vanilla extract. Set to the side.

In another bowl, mix together the almond flour, erythritol, salt, baking powder, nutmeg, cinnamon, and ginger. Set to the side.

Using a cheesecloth or paper towel, take the zucchini and squeeze out the excess water.

Then, whisk the zucchini into the bowl with the eggs.

Slowly add the dry ingredients into the egg mixture using a hand mixer until fully blended.

Lightly spray a 9x5 loaf pan, and spoon in the zucchini bread mixture.

Then, spoon in the chopped walnuts on top of the zucchini bread. Press walnuts into the batter using a spatula.

Bake for 60-70 minutes at 350°F or until the walnuts on top look browned.

KETO PUMPKIN BREAD

With warm spices and crunchy nuts, this keto bread recipe packs your favorite fall flavors into one loaf. Pumpkin and keto flours create a moist and tender base for warm spices like cloves and ginger. Each slice is 3 net carbs — and to stay Bulletproof, simply use grass-fed butter and skip the nutmeg.

Total time: 55min

Serves: 10

INGREDIENTS

- ✓ 1/2 cup butter, softened
- ✓ 2/3 cup erythritol sweetener, like Swerve
- ✓ 4 eggs large
- ✓ 3/4 cup pumpkin puree, canned (see notes for fresh)
- ✓ 1 tsp. vanilla extract
- ✓ 1 1/2 cup almond flour
- ✓ 1/2 cup coconut flour
- ✓ 4 tsp baking powder
- ✓ 1 tsp cinnamon
- ✓ 1/2 tsp. nutmeg
- ✓ 1/4 tsp. ginger

✓ 1/8 tsp. cloves

✓ 1/2 tsp. salt

INSTRUCTIONS

Preheat the oven to 350°F. Grease a 9"x5" loaf pan, and line with parchment paper.

In a large mixing bowl, cream the butter and sweetener together until light and fluffy.

Add the eggs, one at a time, and mix well to combine.

Add the pumpkin puree and vanilla, and mix well to combine.

In a separate bowl, stir together the almond flour, coconut flour, baking powder, cinnamon, nutmeg, ginger, cloves, salt. Break up any lumps of almond flour or coconut flour.

Add the dry ingredients to the wet ingredients, and stir to combine. (Optionally, add up to 1/2 cup of mix-ins, like chopped nuts or chocolate chips.)

Pour the batter into the prepared loaf pan. Bake for 45 - 55 minutes, or until a toothpick inserted into the center of the loaf comes out clean.

If the bread is browning too quickly, you can cover the pan with a piece of aluminum foil.

NOTES

Want to use your own homemade puréed pumpkin? If it's thinner than canned pumpkin, try to remove some of the water to prevent soggy pumpkin bread.

Want cream cheese frosting? Check the post above for an easy cream cheese frosting recipe.

Want some nuts or chocolate chips? Feel free to add 1/2 cup of mix-ins to the batter before baking

Want pumpkin muffins instead? Divide the batter into greased muffin tins. Be sure to reduce the baking time.

LOW-CARB BLUEBERRY ENGLISH MUFFIN BREAD LOAF

Make the most of seasonal blueberries with this sweet and summery keto bread. Using nut butter and almond flour, this recipe creates a crisp crust and muffin-like interior with 3 net carbs per slice. To keep it more Bulletproof, use raw almond or cashew butter and grass-fed butter or ghee, plus swap almond milk with full-fat canned coconut milk.

Total time: 1hr

Serves: 12

INGREDIENTS

- ✓ 1/2 cup almond butter or cashew or peanut butter
- ✓ 1/4 cup butter ghee or coconut oil
- ✓ 1/2 cup almond flour
- ✓ 1/2 tsp. salt
- ✓ 2 tsp. baking powder
- ✓ 1/2 cup almond milk unsweetened
- ✓ 5 eggs beaten
- ✓ 1/2 cup blueberries

INSTRUCTIONS

Preheat oven to 350 degrees F.

In a microwavable bowl melt nut butter and butter together for 30 seconds, stir until combined well.

In a large bowl, whisk almond flour, salt and baking powder together. Pour the nut butter mixture into the large bowl and stir to combine.

Whisk the almond milk and eggs together then pour into the bowl and stir well.

Drop in fresh blueberries or break apart frozen blueberries and gently stir into the batter.

Line a loaf pan with parchment paper and lightly grease the parchment paper as well.

Pour the batter into the loaf pan and bake 45 minutes or until a toothpick in center comes out clean.

Cool for about 30 minutes then remove from pan.

Slice and toast each slice before serving.

CINNAMON ALMOND FLOUR BREAD

This keto bread recipe answers your sweet and spicy cravings with a tender loaf made from gluten-free flours and warm cinnamon. Each serving of this bread delivers 7.6 net carbs, but you can cut more carbs with a sweetener like non-GMO erythritol. Stay more Bulletproof with grass-fed ghee and Ceylon cinnamon, plus avoid eating chia or flax too often.

Total time: 40min

Serves: 8

INGREDIENTS

- ✓ 2 cups fine blanched almond flour (I use Bob's Red Mill)

- ✓ 2 tbsp. coconut flour

- ✓ 1/2 tsp. sea salt

- ✓ 1 tsp. baking soda

- ✓ 1/4 cup Flax seed meal or chia meal (ground chia or flaxseed, see notes for how to make your own)

- ✓ 5 Eggs and 1 egg white whisked together

- ✓ 1.5 tsp Apple cider vinegar or lemon juice

- ✓ 2 tbsp. maple syrup or honey

- ✓ 2–3 tbsp. of clarified butter (melted) or Coconut oil; divided. Vegan butter also works

- ✓ 1 tbsp. cinnamon plus extra for topping

- ✓ Optional chia seed to sprinkle on top before baking

INSTRUCTIONS

Preheat oven to 350F. Line an 8×4 bread pan with parchment paper at the bottom and grease the sides.

In a large bowl, mix together your almond flour, coconut flour, salt, baking soda, flaxseed meal or chia meal, and 1/2 tablespoon of cinnamon.

In another small bowl, whisk together your eggs and egg white. Then add in your maple syrup (or honey), apple cider vinegar, and melted butter (1.5 to 2 tbsp.).

Mix wet ingredients into dry. Be sure to remove any clumps that might have occurred from the almond flour or coconut flour.

Pour batter into a your greased loaf pan.

Bake at 350° for 30-35 minutes, until a toothpick inserted into center of loaf comes out clean. Mine too around 35 minutes but I am at altitude.

Remove from and oven.

Next, whisk together the other 1 to 2 tbsp of melted butter (or oil) and mix it with 1/2 tbsp of cinnamon. Brush this on top of your cinnamon almond flour bread.

Cool and serve or store for later.

NOTES

For storage, it's best to keep wrapped in foil or ziplock in fridge. The bread freezes well for meal prep.

If you you use a larger pan, the loaf slices will be less fluffy but equally delicious.

To make the flaxseed or chia meal, simply place the the flaxseeds or chia seeds in a coffee grinder and grind until a fine meal is formed.

KETO CHOCOLATE ZUCCHINI BREAD

Rich cocoa powder, coconut cream, and low-glycemic sweeteners make an addictive, chocolatey take on zucchini bread. Top this loaf with melty chocolate chips, and each slice still fits in your macros with 3.4 net carbs. To stay more Bulletproof, use Ceylon cinnamon.

Total time: 1hr

Serves: 12

INGREDIENTS

Dry Ingredients

- ✓ 1 1/2 cup almond flour (170g)
- ✓ 1/4 cup unsweetened cocoa powder (25g)
- ✓ 1 1/2 teaspoon baking soda
- ✓ 2 teaspoons ground cinnamon
- ✓ 1/4 teaspoon sea salt
- ✓ 1/2 cup sugar free crystal sweetener (Monk fruit or erythritol) (100g) or coconut sugar if refined sugar free

Wet Ingredients

- ✓ 1 cup zucchini, finely grated measure packed, discard juice/liquid if there is some - about 2 small zucchini

- ✓ 1 large egg

- ✓ 1/4 cup + 2 tablespoon canned coconut cream 100ml

- ✓ 1/4 cup extra virgin coconut oil , melted, 60ml

- ✓ 1 teaspoon vanilla extract

- ✓ 1 teaspoon apple cider vinegar

Filling - Optional

- ✓ 1/2 cup sugar free chocolate chips

- ✓ 1/2 cup chopped walnuts or nuts you like

INSTRUCTIONS

Preheat oven to 180C (375F). Line a baking loaf pan (9 inches x 5 inches) with parchment paper. Set aside.

Remove both extremity of the zucchinis, keep skin on.

Finely grate the zucchini using a vegetable grater. Measure the amount needed in a measurement cup. Make sure you press/pack them firmly for a precise measure and to squeeze out any liquid from the grated zucchini, I usually don't have any! If you do, discard the liquid or keep for another recipe.

In a large mixing bowl, stir all the dry ingredients together: almond flour, unsweetened cocoa powder, sugar free crystal sweetener, cinnamon, sea salt and baking soda. Set aside.

Add all the wet ingredients into the dry ingredients : grated zucchini, coconut oil, coconut cream, vanilla, egg, apple cider vinegar.

Stir to combine all the ingredients together.

Stir in the chopped nuts and sugar free chocolate chips.

Transfer the chocolate bread batter into the prepared loaf pan.

Bake 50 - 55 minutes, you may want to cover the bread loaf with a piece of foil after 40 minute to avoid the top to darken too much, up to you.

The bread will stay slightly moist in the middle and firm up after fully cool down.

COOL DOWN

Cool down 10 minutes in the loaf pan, then cool down on a cooling rack until it reach room temperature. It can take 4 hours as it is a thick bread. Don't slice the bread before it reaches room temperature. If too hot in the center, it will be too soft and fall apart when you slice it. For a faster result, cool down 40 minutes at room temperature, then pop into the fridge for 1 hour. The fridge will create an extra fudgy texture and the bread will be even easier to slice as it firms up.

Store in the fridge up to 4 days in a cake bowl or other airtight container.

GLUTEN-FREE CRANBERRY BREAD

Using a blend of stevia, erythritol, and fresh cranberries, this keto bread strikes the perfect balance between sweet and tart flavors. Plus, this recipe doesn't skimp on berries — it uses an entire 12-ounce bag — and still keeps net carbs down to 5 grams per serving. To keep every bite Bulletproof, use grass-fed butter and omit the molasses.

Total time: 1hr 25min

Serves: 12

INGREDIENTS

- ✓ 2 cups almond flour

- ✓ 1/2 cup powdered erythritol or Swerve, see Note

- ✓ 1/2 teaspoon Steviva stevia powder see Note

- ✓ 1 1/2 teaspoons baking powder

- ✓ 1/2 teaspoon baking soda

- ✓ 1 teaspoon salt

- ✓ 4 tablespoons unsalted butter melted (or coconut oil)

- ✓ 1 teaspoon blackstrap molasses optional (for brown sugar flavor)

- ✓ 4 large eggs at room temperature

- ✓ 1/2 cup coconut milk

✓ 1 bag cranberries 12 ounces

INSTRUCTIONS

Preheat oven to 350 degrees; grease a 9-by-5 inch loaf pan and set aside.

In a large bowl, whisk together flour, erythritol, stevia, baking powder, baking soda, and salt; set aside.

In a medium bowl, combine butter, molasses, eggs, and coconut milk.

Mix dry mixture into wet mixture until well combined.

Fold in cranberries. Pour batter into prepared pan.

Bake until a toothpick inserted in the center of the loaf comes clean, about 1 hour and 15 minutes.

Transfer pan to a wire rack; let bread cool 15 minutes before removing from pan.

Notes:

Sweeteners can be replaced with about 3/4 to 1 cup of any low carb sugar replacement depending on the sweetness desired.

Do not go yet; One last thing to do

If you enjoyed this book or found it useful I'd be very grateful if you'd post a short review on Amazon. Your support really does make a difference. I read all the reviews personally so I can get your feedback and make this book even better.

Thanks again for your support!